Healthcare Reborn

Healthcare Reborn

✦

Innovative Essays That Will Lower Costs and Improve Well Being Through Balance and Harmony

Ram Ramprasad

Writers Club Press
San Jose New York Lincoln Shanghai

Healthcare Reborn
Innovative Essays That Will Lower Costs and Improve Well Being Through Balance and Harmony

Writers Club Press
an imprint of iUniverse, Inc.

For information address:
iUniverse, Inc.
5220 S. 16th St., Suite 200
Lincoln, NE 68512
www.iuniverse.com

ISBN: 0-595-24167-0

Printed in the United States of America

I dedicate this book to the healing of the earth. The healing of the earth will heal our health.

Contents

Acknowledgment

The two individuals who edited this book are Jennifer Wohlwend and Dan Thornton. I owe them my gratitude. Their comments and corrections have shaped this book. Thank you again for all your help.

Introduction

Politicians, employers, healthcare organizations, physicians and consumers are all struggling to find solutions to the high cost of healthcare in America. There are no simple solutions. American enterprise and creativity have, thus far, increased healthcare costs. While in several other industries costs are decreasing, healthcare costs continue to rise. Nobody knows for certain whether costs will increase or decrease in the post-gnomic era, however, most people place their bets on further cost increases due to a spate of new technological breakthroughs and a change in demographics.

The objective of this book is to stir the imagination of the government, business enterprises, educational institutions, healthcare organizations, and the consumer to explore some innovative ideas and strategies that could significantly lower our healthcare costs through a bottoms-up rather than a top-down approach. Large-scale problems do, of course, require large-scale thinking and efforts. But they should never be divorced from the sometimes inconvenient specificity of particulars, the micro (the bottoms-up) aspects that add long-term value to health.

The inter-relationships between the different components of healthcare are almost mind-boggling. Therefore, I have chosen to break down this book into a list of essays on innovation, strategy, reform, and vision. The suggested approaches are in a broad, yet limited variety of areas. Some of these approaches or innovations may already exist. However, some others that are suggested are my own and are specified as such where appropriate. Collectively, I have tried to synthesize them in an effort to address comprehensive solutions to reshape healthcare, lower costs, or in certain cases look at healthcare from a different perspective than the ones we are already familiar with.

The ideas in this book are oriented to the society at large with an aim to benefit the consumer. Medicine and health have always been an expression for human compassion. The more we remember this, the more honest our intentions will be towards health and our ability to lower costs.

Although societal interests are at the heart of these essays, the emphasis on the consumer does not absolve one of his or her personal responsibility or accountability. All innovations make us more accountable and as a society it places on us the onus of being more involved and watchful of our welfare. Every essay challenges us to more closely look at the ramifications of our innovations. Some of the essays call for more direction from our leaders and the government. Even if this direction comes in the form of self-imposed discipline, we some-times thank ourselves in the long run. Therefore, the book advocates certain tax incentives, but also urges government to impose taxes on certain other things. The suggestions need to be treated as "small-scale experiments." The book touches on controversial issues such as Medi-care with an approach to suggest direction and provide innovative options. We simply cannot depend on our children or their children to keep Medicare solvent. My approach seeks a balance that is fair and just to all parties. When we remove balance and ethics from a system, it encourages lopsided growth that is more deleterious than helpful to healthcare in the long run. There are several other strategies and inno-vative options listed in this book that seek to provide a balance that is fair and equitable for all parties.

For corporate organizations, the book proposes several different ways of looking at their businesses. In the opinion of the author, these innovative approaches encourage social entrepreneurship. Healthcare businesses need to operate like true businesses, they need to live within their means and grow within their means. However, corporations also need to constantly challenge themselves on how closely they are con-nected to their vision.

The vision of this book is to seek efficiencies to contain healthcare costs through strategy, reform, and innovation. The book offers innovative solutions that the government, industry, and private individuals can capitalize on to improve the overall quality of life while lowering healthcare costs. Nobody knows what things will look like; systems are an amalgam of a variety of thoughts and actions that churn in a cauldron of a universal mind pool and are balanced by both positive and negative emotions. I have made an attempt in a small way to reconnect the faith we have in our system and our citizens. The more we keep the total wellbeing of an individual and his environment in mind, the better off we will be as a nation. Medicine and health must begin with the right intentions, right ethics, and positive reinforcement to society.

Most of the increases in our healthcare costs can be contained not by research; rather they can be contained in the way we think, the way we connect with our fellow human beings, and the way we protect our environment. Society may need to recognize a collective human purpose; it must then connect the individuals of the society through the principles of free markets to such a purpose. This is the theme of the book and this is the idea in which innovations for the future should follow regardless of which industrial category they belong to. When we approach humanity with the right intention and compassion, our thoughts and research proceed accordingly. This book shows that increases in healthcare costs are not the sole responsibility of any single institution, it is a complex miasma where every industry, society, and the nation are involved. Solutions must be developed with an approach that seeks balance and harmony for everyone in the healthcare marketplace.

It is not the intention of this book to provide a canned solution for the issues related to healthcare, for there may not be one. All I offer are ideas and opinions for the betterment of healthcare through some small-scale experiments. Society and individuals will sort out the rest, they will seek out the right modalities of treatment, a system and a strategy should foster what individuals try to seek out. These individuals know how to control their own destiny and most often they figure out what is right for them. All we have to learn is to observe and create an infrastructure that addresses their innate desires and needs.

The book has four parts and two chapters to each part. **The first chapter of each part is a theoretical narrative interspersed with several unique and creative ideas. The second chapter is a practical application of some of these ideas. When theory and practice are combined it provides direction and an approach to a solution.**

Part 1: Chapter 1 discusses the role of preventive health and offers some unique and innovative ideas on how we need to approach research in preventive health. This chapter also offers some creative ideas on converting the theoretical aspects of preventive health into practical ideas that will benefit society. Chapter 2 offers an innovative idea on converting the Medicaid Food Stamp program into an experiment in preventive health.

Part 2: Chapter 3 offers a vision and recommends a national strategy that may need to be adopted in order to lower healthcare costs for our nation. Chapter 4 predicts how different portable technologies will reshape healthcare.

Part 3: Chapter 5 discusses innovations in reform in several areas such as medical school training, patent laws, death and dying, etc., that will reshape healthcare and lower costs. Chapter 6 is a detailed discussion on Medicare with some new ideas and strategies on how we can make Medicare solvent for years to come.

Part 4: Chapter 7 is a discussion on stress and its association to healthcare costs and how various institutions and organizational design concepts may increase our healthcare costs. The chapter also discusses how our educational system may be contributing to increased stress in society. Identified in this chapter are some examples of social innovations that may help society address the high cost of healthcare. Chapter 8 offers several unique ideas for policy makers and to corporations to establish a vision based on ideals which nurture the environment. A true ideal creates true progress. In the long run, it is ideals alone that will lower healthcare costs.

I have deliberately chosen not to discuss much detail in the introduction since this has a tendency for the cursory reader to form conclusions without reading the book. Although the book is written in an essay style, **readers are encouraged to read the book from cover to cover** since chapters are interrelated and the flow of logic is in sequence. Independent reading of each chapter may at times provide a different takeaway message and that is not the intention of this book. The opinions mentioned in this book are solely of the author.

PART I

1

Innovations in Preventive Health

The way we age depends less on who we are than on how we live—what we eat, how much we exercise and how we employ our minds. The increase in the rate of diabetes and various other cardiovascular diseases is clear evidence that most Americans do less exercise than in previous generations. As a nation, we are more eager to spend an enormous amount of our healthcare dollars in our health breakdown rather than on health prevention.

Respected studies have shown that exercise can ward off several diseases. Experts now agree that most of the physical decline that older people suffer stems not from age, but from simple neglect. Exercise can preserve and revive most of our health. In a landmark 1986 study, Dr. Ralph Paffenbarger showed that for 19,000 participants in his study, the death rates fell in direct proportion to the number of calories burned each week.[1] It is not just exercise, but also what we eat plays a major role in our health. In controlled studies, San Francisco cardiologist Dr. Dean Ornish has shown that a diet based on low-fat, nutrient-rich foods not only prevents heart disease, but also can help reverse it.[2] Other studies suggest that dietary changes could virtually eliminate the high blood pressure that puts 50 million older Americans at high risk for stroke, heart attack and kidney failure.[3] The age-reversing effects of a plant-based diet are not in question. When you subsist mainly on fresh plant foods, as our ancestors did for roughly seven million years, you get 10 times more potassium than sodium. We need to correct sev-

9

eral of our modern day imbalances that encourage a more sedentary lifestyle by providing incentives in our economic system for people to make healthy changes in their lifestyles.

According to Dr. Karl-Otto Liebmann, Associate Clinical Professor of Psychiatry at Yale University School of Medicine, "The time has come for the eating public to face a stark reality: The consumption of food, if allowed to grow at the present rate, will bankrupt our great nation. Production of food has risen from 10 percent to more than 30 percent of the gross domestic product since 1945. The Congressional Budget Office estimates that by the year 2010 Americans will spend more money and time on eating than on working, vacationing, and being sick combined."[4] It is time that individuals, the government and the healthcare industry took action to provide positive incentives to change behavior. The following is a list of suggestions that can correct the imbalances in our system through the implementation of tax incentives.

ENCOURAGING RESEARCH THAT MAY LOWER THE COSTS OF PREVENTIVE HEALTH

Two of America's most widely read medical journals neglect disease prevention in their published research studies, say scientists at Virginia Commonwealth University.[5] According to their report in the August issue of *The American Journal of Preventive Medicine*, both *The New England Journal of Medicine* and *The Journal of American Medical Association* preferentially publish research on treatment of specific diseases instead of studies emphasizing the importance of preventive measures. Researchers examined all investigations, reviews, editorials, and special reports published in the two journals during 1998. Only 71—or six percent—of the 1,160 articles focused on disease prevention. In addition, only 11 articles focused on diet, exercise, and other health-promoting behaviors.[6]

One way to increase our focus on prevention is to encourage the scientific community to publish more research articles on prevention. For example, how many research articles exist on the effects of computer screen radiation, or television screen radiation on eye health or on pregnant women? These studies are scattered or almost non-existent. Similarly, do we know the effects of cell phone use and its link with cancer? Some people believe that the constant impact of radio waves from cell phones may cause certain tumors in the brain. If there are established links, then what are the solutions? Do we have research in these areas of preventive health? If they do exist, why have they not become mainstream?

Should industrial companies come out with a new and less damaging invention of a computer screen, TV screen, or cell phone? Research dollars should automatically flow on the study of the benefits of these inventions if there were found to be some correlation to better eye health or cancer prevention. It is surprising that this kind of research never precedes novel inventions.

Ideas and inventions are geared mostly towards finding a cure at the end point of a disease. I do not argue that the value of finding a cure at the end stage of a disease is less important than prevention. Rather, I argue that institutions must find ways to fund more research projects towards prevention rather than on the control, symptomatic relief, or cure of a disease. If both industry and research institutions follow parallel paths in research, our solutions to healthcare problems will only be delayed. This is well evidenced by the amount of research papers that flood the market on a similar topic, such as, the benefits of Drug XYZ for hypertensive patients. According to Randy Scott, Chief Scientific Officer, Incyte Genomics, 70 to 80 percent of medical research is wasted because graduate students and postdocs repeat past experiments as part of their training, and scientists refuse to share their research until it's published, which can be up to two years after the results are compiled.[7]

Achieving diversity in healthcare research is paramount for achieving overall reductions in healthcare costs. When research is focused on a singular path or theme, we lose sight of treatment options that could have provided similar outcomes. For example, a low-cost research project to determine the health effects of sleeping in sync with the magnetic poles of the earth could result in surprising outcomes.

In ancient India, traditional physicians used a method called 'pulse diagnosis' to accurately diagnose diseases within the human body. It was believed that, just like radio signals, the pulse emits different frequencies or signals. Each frequency or signal was associated with a specific disease. Although this practice is now extinct, research could lead to the implementation of diagnostic equipment capable of performing this function.

Similarly, in some developing countries, people brush their teeth with their finger and toothpowder. One could hypothesize that toothpowder, due its dry nature, removes plaque in a better manner than toothpaste. Also, brushing with a finger may cause fewer traumas to the gum than brushing with a toothbrush. Brushing with a finger may provide better and vigorous massage to the gums, without causing trauma. Researchers are now exploring how bacteria in the mouth may be associated with many health conditions, including diabetes, cardiovascular disease, pre-term births, and strokes. On the surface, this suggestion may sound bizarre. It is important to understand, however, the philosophical basis of the cultures that adopted these methods.

If researchers were aware of behavior in other cultures, we would have seen toothbrushes and toothpaste that mimic the properties of a finger and the toothpowder respectively. I am not advocating that we change our habits in this country, but rather am trying to make a point on better prevention. Cultures of most developing countries could improve their dental health by using dental floss. Preventive health is an ideal mix of technology, instinct, awareness, and science. Learning from other cultures, learning from animals and their instincts (see Chapter 3), and a judicious use of technology could create better models of preventive health. Research and simple innovations in the area of preventive dental health can save us an enormous amount of costs in healthcare.

These ideas may sound radical, but who is to say that adopting this thought process will not reduce healthcare costs? The most important research results are not necessarily correlated with the amount of money spent on the study. Such results are based on the way we think with open mindedness and societal interests at heart. Einstein used "thought experiments," and Edison used his garage, to develop some of the world's greatest inventions. Poor countries have developed their own low-cost methods for affordable healthcare, as noted above. For example, as mentioned previously, countries have achieved good dental health while avoiding toothbrushes, toothpaste, and several other associated gadgets. More prosperous countries have gone about it in a different manner. However, all of these countries could have benefited one another by developing an optimal mix that could be tailored to the specific cultural nuances of each country.

The example above does not demonstrate that there are superior and inferior roles in research, nor does it prove that low-cost or high-cost research provides the best solutions. We should not judge, but rather have an open mind. People all over the world have found unique ways to arrive at solutions for healthcare. This is the reason why America needs to encourage diversity in research with an open attitude to different schools of thought and cultural behaviors. If our real desire is to reduce healthcare costs, we should be open to explore all schools of philosophy of medicine. In particular, we need to pay special attention to where research findings resulted in the efficient use of resources and reduced overall costs.

It is troubling that both managed care and the health industry spend more time and effort on creating programs that manage diseases rather than on programs that prevent health. Fortunately, the widespread use of the Internet seems to be slowly changing this paradigm. Few managed care companies have ventured to be creative in the area of preventive health. Most preventive health efforts have been in the area of public education materials and campaigns.

We do not hear of a joint venture between a hi-tech company and a Health Maintenance Organization (HMO). These organizations could have collaborated to create a television or a computer screen that does not damage our eyes or does not have an adverse effect on pregnant women. A cell phone company could collaborate with an HMO to find out whether there is a link between cell phone use and cancer. If there is a link, a cell phone company will not lose all sales. On the contrary, the findings would provide the cell phone company with a first mover advantage in the quest to develop a new technology based on its research. Research partnerships among companies in dissimilar fields is one way of reducing the costs of healthcare. Companies will grow if they anticipate the effects of their inventions on society, the environment, and on human health. Companies should be open to hiring or establishing departments that specialize in healthcare anthropology.

Many developing countries still use leaded gas because they cannot afford to buy unleaded gas. The rate of asthma in these countries is extremely high. Yet, research on how to reduce reliance on gasoline do not become a priority until gas prices increase significantly. When the outcome of every invention incorporates the ultimate benefit to society, all parties benefit. Sharp increases in healthcare costs may be the result of corporate actions or "progress." For instance, Mark Lipson, Policy Program Director, Organic Farming Research Foundation, points to organic tortilla chip maker Terra Prima, which had to recall 87,000 bags of its chips after tests by a Netherlands-based distributor found that they contained genetically modified corn.[8] Farmers can't sell crops that have genetically modified pollen blown by the wind onto their fields because of the uncertainty of the health effect of corn with recombinant DNA. No one really knows effects these crops would have on our health or how will they increase our healthcare costs.

According to scientists studying coral reefs, fully a quarter of world's coral reefs have effectively died due to global warming.[9] Coral reefs are a potential source for medical innovations like joint and bone replacement. Marine biologists have established a connection between global warming and the bleaching of corals. However, our understanding and research between the linkages of climatological and ecological change as determinants of public health is lagging. According to Dr. Jonathan Patz, Department of Occupational & Environmental Medicine, Johns Hopkins University, " Addressing this newly recognized threat will require interdisciplinary cooperation among health professionals, climatologists, biologists, and social scientists, and will necessitate research beyond conventional dose-response linear relationships to address complex systems-based ecological processes."[10] Malaria and dengue fever serve as prime examples of climate-sensitive diseases. Climate-related increases in sea surface temperature could lead to a higher incidence of water-based cholera and shellfish poisoning. Ozone, a result of global warming, is a harmful pollutant and can damage lung tissue. This list of adverse health effects of global warming goes on and on, and includes even skin cancer. The World Health Organization considers global warming a serious public health challenge of the future. Public health initiatives must minimize the ill effects of our actions, before any grand research provides a rude awakening. We must not wait until nature teaches us a tough lesson and humble our intellect. Our total reliance on proof, data, and research has diminished our emotional intelligence and reliance on the use of basic common sense.

Few, if any, hi-tech companies evaluate the effects of their inventions on health. Government and policy makers can play a role in this area by offering incentives for companies who incorporate preventive health measures in their inventions. Had this been the norm, we would have come out with hybrid cars before Toyota or Honda. History has proven that what works for the customer and the environment—the total well-being of an individual and his surroundings—always wins and tends to capture a greater share in the marketplace. Customers may not be sure in the beginning of how their lives will be affected by a particular product or service, but they ultimately figure these things out. As a matter of fact, consumers are sometimes willing to pay a premium for these products and services. This is one reason why disruptive technologies may pose a threat to established technologies.

Universities strapped for money and grants are better off promoting low cost research. As long as the intentions are sincere on helping humanity, low-cost or high-cost research, the results could be the same. When all research is focused on the next "hot" field, motives may be confused and researchers may pursue the field in search of a quick financial reward. For example, the Human Genome project promises a detailed map of the genetic landscape. In a way, it is a rather prosaic step, but what lies beyond is breathtaking. However, if every organization depended on the Human Genome for all of their answers, then intentions would be questionable. About 98 percent of our illnesses are environmental and behavioral and not necessarily genetic. As a society, we need to determine how we allocate our resources. Diversity in research, genuine intentions to find the right answers, and the right allocation of resources as a society will help us achieve reductions in total healthcare costs.

INNOVATIONS IN TAX INCENTIVES FOR PEOPLE WHO EXERCISE

Federal and State governments can play a crucial role in promoting preventive healthcare through some small-scale experiments. The Surgeon General's 1996 report on "Physical Activity and Health" states that nearly half of all 12 to 21 year olds are not regularly physically active, and that by age 19, about 38 percent of males and 51 percent of females are not even moderately physically active.[11]

In order to combat this lack of physical activity the Government should provide tax exemptions for people who exercise. The following is a description of how the government would administer such a program. All exercise equipment would be equipped with a timing device. When a person is ready to exercise, he or she would scan an encrypted card in this machine and scan the card out when he or she is finished exercising. The card would electronically capture the individuals total time of exercise. Simple and portable electronic card scanners would enable one to keep track of the number of hours they exercise. At the time of filing tax returns, individuals would claim the appropriate tax exemptions for the number of hours they had exercised. Innovative companies would figure out how to create these machines for various fitness equipment including newly manufactured as well as existing equipment. The companies would also determine how to create these gadgets for joggers, swimmers, and various other outdoor exercise enthusiasts. Each individual would have his or her own card. This would encourage people to exercise anywhere: in their own home, outdoors, fitness centers, or in a fitness center provided by their employer.

Should the government fail to act on this suggestion, private healthcare companies would have a unique opportunity to provide frequent flyer airline credit miles for the number of hours the individual exercises. HMOs or other major healthcare or pharmaceutical companies could manufacture these "exercise frequent flyer cards," and market them to individuals. These companies can then work with the Federal Government to allow people to set aside tax free dollars in their medical savings accounts for the number of hours that was spent on exercise. In this manner, private enterprise can take steps to transform and create a social culture that believes in preventive health through monetary incentives. Although the current healthcare system exhibited a great deal of creativity, the system has yet to develop unique monetary incentives. However, we have lacked in developing unique monetary incentives that promote health. We need to stretch capitalism to social innovations to contain costs.

Under such a program small, medium, and large companies would be encouraged to open more fitness centers for employees to exercise. Similar to some mandatory requirements like training programs, employees may be required to log in a minimum of 30-50 hours of exercise per year, regardless of location. Government would provide tax credits for individuals and the industry for the number of exercise hours that are logged in on a per-employee basis. Individuals would claim tax exemptions for the number of exercise hours they logged in. These could be easily tracked through the suggested time card system.

Consider these 1996 studies on fitness:

- GE Aircraft employees who used the company's fitness center for three years cut their average annual healthcare costs from $1,044 to $757 per person. In contrast, non-member costs increased from $773 to $941 per person.[12]

- Physically active employees at Mesa Petroleum Company spent $217 less on medical claims annually per person and took 21 fewer hours of sick time than did sedentary employees.[13]

Shannon Entin, a publisher and editor of *Fitness Link*, recommends tax rebates on the purchase of fitness equipment. She also reports that the IRS recently responded to a 58-page letter from the American Obesity Association requesting a deduction for weight management programs. The IRS sought evidence that effective weight management contributes to corporate profits before offering such a deduction. What the IRS may not be aware of is that since the 1970s there has been a fivefold increase in the esophageal cancer known as adenocarcinoma, which is not clearly associated with alcohol or tobacco. Among white males, the incidence of this formerly rare tumor has risen more rapidly than any other cancer.[14] Possible factors cited for this rise include reflux caused by an epidemic of obesity, increased dietary fat and the reflux-producing effects of some new medicines.

However, if we leave these issues to manufacturers to invent the type of device I suggest we can rest assured that industry will take the initiative to find a tax incentive for the public. Purchasing fitness machines is not in and of itself a guarantee that people will exercise, therefore, the government may not provide tax incentives on a purchase. It is hard to argue against a membership in a gymnasium. Money is the single biggest motivator that can change behavior.

ENCOURAGING PREVENTIVE HEALTH THROUGH FOOD SUBSIDY PROGRAMS

Companies should be encouraged to subsidize healthy foods in company-run cafeterias while offsetting the decrease by increasing the cost of unhealthy foods. Research has shown that people develop their eating habits from childhood. As such, while the private industry adopts all of these techniques, the federal government also should start a similar scheme through the $6 billion lunch programs in our country's public schools. If we are accustomed to eating junk food as small children, the greater likelihood that we continue these habits when we become older. It is no coincidence that the world's production of sugarcane for the year 2000 was nearly 1.3 billion metric tons, more than the total production of wheat and rice combined.[15] We teach the concepts of a food pyramid in schools all across America. The irony is that we live in a world where we have reversed the food pyramid. We then debate the macro-rhetoric on the causes of diabetes. The immutable laws on the costs associated with "breakdown" versus "preventive" maintenance have never changed. If this law were untrue, then our cars would never need an oil change.

The government may want to consider measures to institute creative healthy food habits in schools across America. Restaurants and fast food chains that offer healthy menu choices should be granted creative tax incentives. As nations' economies grow stronger, tax incentives in the future must shift more towards devising clever and creative ways to induce lifestyle changes. These suggestions will expand and not contract the economy.

The Federal Government should also encourage food manufacturers to develop an improved formula for the "nutrition facts" labels that are listed on the back of most processed food packaging. By the time a consumer reads or has the time to read the nutrition facts and decipher all of the nutritional content such as amount of fat, cholesterol, sodium, potassium, etc., the consumer is left confused and bewildered. All nutrition fact labels should have a simple preventive health index that could have a letter grading between "A" through "D," so that both children and adults would relate to this versus their place in the food pyramid. For example, on one extreme, red meats and certain canned foods would have a "D" grade and natural juices an "A" grade. Beverages with aspartame may have a different grade, like "N" for neutral indication or a grade that implies controversies associated with an ingredient such as aspartame. This strategy may provide the government a choice to tax "D" grade food items and divert consumers towards healthy foods and ultimately induce a change in behavior.

It is possible that the government may not have considered letter grading due to the negative connotations on calling food, "good" or "bad" since all food is valuable and can support life. It is the degree of consumption or the reversal of the food pyramid that we follow that leads consumers towards unhealthy eating habits. In this sense, the letter grading may only be appropriate for purposes of creating different levels of taxes.

THE URGENCY TO PROVIDE TAX INCENTIVES FOR PREVENTIVE HEALTH

Heart disease, cancer, strokes and other leading lifestyle-related maladies have emerged as the leading causes of death and disability. According to the National Center for Health Statistics, the majority of U.S. deaths are caused by destructive lifestyles, such as smoking, eating a poor diet, and physical inactivity. Unfortunately, Western nations are exporting diseases of affluence to their global neighbors.

By the year 2020—unless significant public health changes occur—heart disease, severe depression, traffic accidents, stroke and chronic lung diseases will be the leading causes of disability in the world. According to the World Health Organization and the World Bank, the table below is the anticipated shift that will happen in 2020 with respect to major disease conditions. Therefore, it is important that we tie monetary incentives to preventive health strategies. We have used interest rate policies to contain inflation and recession, therefore, we may want to utilize similar policies to affect a change in lifestyle.

Rank	1990	2020
1	Pneumonia	Heart Disease
2	Diarrheal diseases	Severe depression
3	Diseases of the newborn	Traffic accidents
4	Severe depression	Stroke
5	Heart disease	Chronic lung disease

CONCLUSION

The United States has the highest expenditures for healthcare in the world. We spend more than 14 percent of our GNP on healthcare. It behooves the Government to shift its tax and economic policies to change behavior on these issues through creative tax incentive schemes. This is taking economics to a new level, while increasing innovation and employment in the country.

Economists could argue that tax incentives are inappropriate to induce lifestyle changes. From a purely economic perspective, one could even argue that healthcare costs for the nation as a whole would not be reduced if people were to die young or old. This is not true. It is to the benefit of the economy to make people live longer and healthier.

The longer and healthier people live, the fewer healthcare dollars a nation would spend. Researchers have found that the oldest of the old often enjoy better health than people in their 70s.[16] The 79 centenarians in Perls's New England Study have all lived independently through their early 90s, taking an average of just one medication. Moreover, when the time comes for these hearty souls to die, they do not linger. In a 1995 study, James Lubitz of the Health Care Financing Administration calculated that medical expenditures for the last two years of life—statistically the most expensive—average $22,600 for people who die at 70, but just $8,300 for those who make it past 100.[17] This proves the point that the longer and healthier people live, the lower the total healthcare costs. Therefore, offering monetary and tax incentives may reduce healthcare costs for the country while providing overall quality-of-life benefits to humanity. It is also recommended that research in healthcare be diverse and encourage a pluralistic vision to reduce the overall costs of healthcare.

Similar to the Internet, the computer, and the technological revolution, the United States could again be at the forefront of developing a preventive health model that could become the envy of the world.

2

The Medicaid Food Stamp Program—A Novel Experiment in Preventive Health

T he link between diet and health has been accepted and is now published in several scientific publications. Magazines on health and prevention often talk about the relationship between diet and exercise. Unfortunately, to date, no institution or company may have combined with one another to assess the health of an individual based solely on his food consumption. The Federal government, through its Medicaid food stamp program, has the opportunity to form a partnership and create a new organization with the help of pharmacy benefit management companies, grocery store chains, and food manufacturers. The opportunity or idea outlined below would create a win-win situation for both public and private institutions.

It is estimated that government food stamp program expenditures total approximately $12 billion on an annual basis, allowing over 18 million people to buy groceries.[1] Of this total, the Department of Agriculture and Federal Bureau of Investigation estimate that over $1.8 billion is lost due to procedural errors and acts of fraud.[2] Thousands of low-income families have been unable to obtain benefits worth millions of dollars because of these inefficiencies. Additionally, the inefficient manner in which participants spend the allotted food stamp dollars –the first week the recipient dines on lobster but lives without food stamps for the remaining eligibility period—has been well documented in various press and government publications. A combination of program inefficiencies, fraud and aberrant consumption creates patterns that often result in the poor nutrition, and therefore the poor health of program recipients. These facts have been increasingly exposed by the press, seriously embarrassing the federal and state governments.[3]

Healthcare companies, managed care organizations, and pharmacy benefit management companies have a unique opportunity to change this paradigm through the development of a program that supports "Appropriate Diet Care" for the 20 million people enrolled in the food stamp program. The link between diet and health is unchallenged. These are some quotes from well-known associations:

"It is the position of The American Dietetic Association that optimal nutrition and physical activity can promote health and reduce the risk of chronic disease."[4]

"The American Cancer Society recommends to: choose most foods from plant sources, limit intake of high-fat foods (particularly from animal source, be physically active, maintain healthy body weight, and limit consumption of alcoholic beverages."[5]

HOW DOES THE PROGRAM WORK?

The Federal government has a unique opportunity to partner with a newly formed organization, which could be established by pharmacy benefit management companies (due to their expertise in this area), HMOs, grocery store chains, and/or food manufacturers. These entities could collaborate and effectively carve out the food stamp program. An effective plan for this development may be the creation of a state-by-state pilot project. Gradually phasing in this project would enable the government to effectively manage the food stamp program project and apply the appropriate information management, cost containment and healthy diet techniques for the food stamp recipients.

The following is how the newly formed organization would build an "Appropriate Diet Care" program for the food stamp recipients:

1. <u>Network Management:</u> Zip codes of the food stamp recipients would be matched to major grocery store chains. The government's industrial partner (the newly formed organization) would contract with the major grocery store chains to administer a pricing reimbursement formula, which would basically be the retail price of the food item minus a percentage discount. Major chain food stores would choose to participate in this program because they will now attract food stamp recipients into their stores. This is similar to pharmacy benefit management companies contracting with pharmacy chains to obtain discounts on pharmaceuticals for participation in a program that their company creates.

2. Preferred or healthy food products would require no cash outlay by the food stamp recipient, and non-preferred or unhealthy food items would require a higher cash outlay. This is again similar to how a pharmacy prescription card works, generic drugs have a lower cash outlay or a copay and brand drugs have a higher cash outlay or a copay.

3. The government and nutrition experts of the newly formed organization would develop an appropriate food formulary for preferred vs. non-preferred food products based on cost, food quality and impact on overall health. Again, this concept is similar to that of the formulary established by health plans or pharmacy benefit management companies.

4. The newly formed organization, on behalf of the government, would obtain rebates from food manufacturers and distributors for the inclusion of their food items on the preferred food formulary list.

5. The newly formed organization would replace food stamps with ID cards similar to a pharmacy prescription drug card.

6. Using the ID card, a point-of-sale technology network would be used by the participating food stores to obtain customer information and covered food products.

7. The point-of-sale technology network could be applied to link both pharmacy and food benefits for the Medicaid/food stamp recipients, thus achieving further efficiencies in integrating the appropriate diet care and the pharmacy prescription card programs.

The above-listed technological and logistical applications already exist and are in use in the pharmacy benefit management industry. The integration of these techniques into the administration of the federal food stamp program has the potential to solve many of the inefficiencies previously discussed. There already appears to be an opportunity for the government and industry to collaborate and apply private business administrative techniques in a bold and novel experiment to address these pressing issues and demonstrate savings in healthcare costs through appropriate diet care concepts.

The advantages of such a modified program would be immense. It would offer the government an opportunity to save money by eliminating inefficiencies through use of a point-of-sale technology network. It would avoid waste and abuse, reduce bureaucracy, foster rebate sharing, generate savings through a discounted network of food chains, and incorporate the advantages of a private enterprise system. The government would be influencing the behavior of food program recipients with an integrated food and pharmacy formulary. Such an integrated food and pharmacy program enables the government and the newly-formed company to closely track the health of its food program recipients from an aggregated perspective.

There are several indirect benefits that would be achieved through the integration of pharmacy benefits into the food program. At the present time, Medicaid receives rebates from the pharmaceutical industry for the medicines that are consumed by Medicaid recipients through its administration of the pharmacy program on a state-by-state basis. In the suggested program, the newly formed company will consolidate all of these state level mechanisms, thus enabling efficiencies for both the government and the pharmaceutical industry. The Pharmaceutical Industry would now only have to work with one company that would be involved in receiving the Medicaid rebates for pharmaceuticals.

The newly formed company would generate a stream of revenue through administrative commissions from the government for rebates that it would collect from the food industry, the pharmaceutical industry, etc. The government saves money through administrative and procedural errors, rebates, and through the sale of data and research to the private sector. The objective of streamlining the Medicaid program is not in the savings. It is in the government vision to reshape healthcare along with the private enterprise system in unique and different ways through the application of food science concepts, information technology, adoption of current pharmaceutical benefit management concepts, etc.

FUTURE APPLICATIONS OF FOOD/PHARMACY BENEFIT MANAGEMENT CONCEPT TO THE PRIVATE SECTOR

The integration of food and pharmacy benefit management concepts could have an application in the private sector, especially for those individuals who already have prescription drug program coverage. Pharmacy benefit management companies and HMOs, in collaboration with grocery store chains with their own in-house pharmacies, can issue food and prescription drug cards to their existing clientele.

Grocery chains could send out statements to individuals regarding food consumption habits for households. This would help families track their consumption habits just like they track their expenses on a phone bill or electricity bill. Grocery stores would now have an ability to benchmark a household's food purchases with an ideal food pyramid or a national benchmark. Grocery store chains could also utilize the data for effective market positioning. For example, a grocery store selling more organic foods could potentially show that their buying population has a lower incidence of disease. This assumes the buying population utilizes the same store for both food and pharmacy purchases. This program would be optional for consumers. It would allow grocery retailers to position their businesses for merchandising food as well as promoting preventive health. At the present time, grocery retailers see their business as merely food distribution. Once they define their business as being "preventive health," their opportunities would expand.

The concept may allow life science and pharmaceutical companies to truly experiment the value of functional foods, neutraceuticals, and biopharmaceuticals by using the grocery store as a sponsor for their clinical trials. This system could make it easier for companies to experiment and obtain a neutraceutical claim on any specific supplement or functional food. Typically, the in-house retail pharmacy of a grocery store would sponsor and monitor the trial. It would empower the role of pharmacists, physicians, and consumers. Ability to combine and integrate data on OTCs, pharmaceuticals and food has the potential of generating new streams of revenue for almost all of the parties involved, to include grocery stores, pharmacy benefits management companies, HMOs, and pharmaceutical manufacturers. The entire area of food and pharmacy benefits integration may serve as a harbinger for several research topics for epidemiologists and scientists, thus enabling them to collectively address healthcare costs in an integrated fashion.

CONCLUSION

A collaborative effort between pharmacy benefit management companies, HMOs, grocery store chains and the government will ultimately prepare us to address the health of Americans in a more systematic and meaningful manner. The evolution of pharmaceutical companies to life science companies, and the suggested potential evolution of grocery store chains, HMOs, and PBMs, to promoters of preventive health may benefit several parties, as well as the population as a whole. In the year, 2010, the Center for Medicaid and Medicare Services (CMS), formerly known as the Health Care Financing Administration (HCFA) estimates that $70 billion will be spent by Medicaid on prescription drugs.[6] I estimate food expenditures for the Medicaid population to reach up to $30 billion for the same time period.[7] This thus represents a $100 billion combined business potential for firms who can step up to the challenge of integrating these benefits for the Medicaid population. Finally, the scenario allows better overall health and more informed consumer choices to the consumer without sacrificing liberty or options.

PART II

3

Innovations in Healthcare Strategy and Implications on Healthcare Costs

Thirty years ago, U.S. national healthcare expenditures averaged $341 per person, per year. For the year 2000, the projected average was $4,611 per person, per year, an increase of 1,352 percent.[1] In terms of real dollars, in 1970 national health expenditures were $73.2 billion, while for the year 2000 the projected number was $1,316.2 billion, an increase of 1,800 percent. The gross domestic product (GDP) in 1970 was $1,035.6 billion and in year 2000 it was about $9,193.8 billion, an increase of 887 percent. From 1970 to 2000, national health expenditures as a percent of GDP grew from 7 percent to 14 percent.[2] The Health Care Financing Administration (now known as Center for Medicaid and Medicare Services –CMS) expects this contribution to reach 16 percent by the year 2008. All of these statistics are available on the **www.HCFA.gov** website.

If you marry the above statistics with those from the National Vital Statistics Report, one may surmise that these high growth rates in healthcare are not sustainable. The average life expectancy in the year 1900 was 47.3 years, growing to 70.8 years in 1970 and to 76.5 years in 1997.[3] In a period of 100 years, we added 30 years in average life expectancy. The first half of the increase in life expectancy was probably more likely due to improvements in public health, sanitation, and finding cures for infectious diseases than to advances in medical care.

According to Dr. Daniel Callahan, cofounder of the Hastings Center and a visiting scholar at Harvard Medical School, the great increase in life expectancy of about 60 percent to 70 percent has come from social and economic factors, and not medical progress.[4] The second half, however, may be the result of unprecedented innovations in medical care. Dr. Callahan, further adds, "To me, the great puzzle in our present situation is why we are so terrific on the technological side—so aggressive, entrepreneurial, imaginative—and yet so regressive on the social side."[5]

With healthcare costs growing at a rate twice that of GDP, there is cause for concern from many individuals. Whether we will experience similar increases in growth rates is hard to predict. The rapid medical and genomic innovations may be the harbinger of further increases in healthcare costs. Also, the U.S. population age 65 and older will increase from 20.9 million in 1970 to 38.4 million in 2008 adding a great burden to our healthcare system.[6]

Now that we have some perspective on healthcare statistics, we need not be alarmed but we do need to feel concerned, because the crisis in healthcare is a real one. We should watch out for further anticipated increases in growth rates for healthcare costs. The global human population is exploding at the rate of 80 million a year, or a billion every twelve years. In the year 1800, there were about a billion people on planet earth, two billion in 1925, three billion in 1960, and about six billion today. However, the U.S. population will not continue to grow at such a rapid pace. For year 2000, our projected population is expected to reach 303.6 million. These increases in population could indirectly increase our healthcare costs. We will see later how this could be so. Factors that we overlook are rarely of concern until people realize later how such factors have affected our society.

Listed below are some innovations in vision and strategy that, if embraced with an open mind, may provide solutions for healthcare issues and high costs.

A PERSPECTIVE ON THE HIGH GROWTH IN OUR HEALTHCARE EXPENDITURES

The key concerns that healthcare economists should identify and examine are the areas that led to the high growth rate of healthcare costs. Trying to critically examine areas that show above average growth rate versus a simulated and a reasonable growth rate might illuminate solutions to the root cause of our problems. All of the appropriate statistics needed for any sophisticated modeling are available on the HCFA website (now CMS). Trying to rely on propaganda and myopic issues are irrelevant in this day and age when information is readily available. Using the data available on the site, one can easily analyze the percentage of our expenses allocated to vision care, dental health, physician services, prescription drugs, and many other areas.

For example, there are several press bulletins. One of these bulletins on the National Institutes of Health website shows that in 1996, the average annual health expenditure was $5,864 for people age 65 through 69, rising to $16,465 at age 85 and older.[7] Obviously, when we try to interpret data on the current average healthcare expenditure of $4,611 for all people, we know that it is skewed more towards the elderly, this is expected. Therefore, one of the key innovations in healthcare is to minimize the high cost for care of the elderly through appropriate and ethical means. However, the statistics do imply that we are more compassionate in our technologies at the end stage of a person's life. It is likely the case that our total healthcare dollars are weighed more towards critical care rather than preventive care. William C. Walters III, MD, in his book *The Grand Disguise*, wonders if it is reasonable that hospital costs have risen 15,000 percent in a half-century with the same number of hospitals and 33 percent fewer beds.[8]

We need to ask ourselves if the increase in technology has overwhelmed our hospitals, and whether it is reasonable for every hospital to have all of the latest technology. Have we ever asked the seniors of the country what it is that they really want from the U.S. healthcare system? Is it more technology or is it more innovation on the social side? While catering to the needs of the elderly through the use of technology, have we over-served the needs of the healthy as well? If the goal of healthcare is to have a healthy and long life with a painless end, can we say that we have provided this for our elderly based on their true and innate desires? (see chapter 5 on Innovations in Reform).

Excluding the fact that average annual healthcare expenditures may be slightly skewed towards the elderly, several other components that contributed to the growth in healthcare may or may not be justifiable. Average life expectancy increased from 47 to 77 years in the last 100 years due to several factors, according to Dr. Callahan. He is right that these factors have contributed to the increase in the average life span. Some of these factors may have included the absence of major and devastating wars after the late 1940s, the influx of immigrants increasing our population base, and the discovery and production of several new medicines, and improvements in public health might have also contributed to the increase in life expectancy.

One modern medical miracle has been the invention of vaccines. Vaccines are one of medicine's bright and shining stars. Before vaccines, parents in the United States could expect that every year polio would paralyze 10,000 children; rubella would cause birth defects and mental retardation in as many as 20,000 newborns; measles would infect about 4 million children and kill several thousands. Diphtheria was one of the most common causes of death in school-aged children. The Hib bacterium would cause meningitis leaving many with permanent brain damage, and pertussis killed 8,000 children.[9] The invention of vaccines in the mid 1950s changed the lives of several million children both in the U.S. and abroad. For example, smallpox has been eradicated throughout the world.

However, with increased life expectancy we now have several new kinds of chronic diseases resulting from old age, such as diabetes, cardiovascular diseases, mental diseases, bone diseases, arthritic diseases, poorer eye and dental health, etc. Each of these chronic diseases, and the slow increase in our aging population, has hastened or spurred several breakthrough innovations in medical care. They relate to delivery of care, diagnostics, more sophisticated hospital comforts, and better medicines. All of these factors are important for our quality of life and every one of them is equally appealing and justifiable. However, the worry is whether we can afford the pace of this growth, especially, if the growth is faster than our paychecks.

Many inventions do improve our quality of life. If laser surgery gives someone the gift of better sight, it is justified. If a certain medicine could save someone from a heart attack, it could be justified. If a flu vaccine allows one to carry out important business duties without falling sick, it is justified. However, if an MRI was used to diagnose an ingrown toenail, the cost would be considered unnecessary, even ridiculous. Similarly, CAT scans and MRIs in general are considered great advancements but are not proven to increase longevity. Therefore, this list can go on and on, and the issues become very complex. We now see a scenario where there was a great retreat of lethal diseases due to nutrition, socio-economic factors, public health and some breakthrough curative medicines. However, the increased longevity has led to chronic illnesses due to a sedentary lifestyle. We have also seen a spate of medical innovations that either give us relief or provided a better quality of life or longevity.

How we contain healthcare costs becomes a matter of perspective. The approach in this book is to offer some ideas that can help contain the pace of growth by changing the way we think and innovate. We can never really contain costs but we certainly can contain the pace of their growth. This is already beginning to happen and will continue its momentum.

The key is to identify inefficiencies in the system and focus on areas that need to grow in line with expectations that are sound, reasonable, and compatible with the various philosophies and the variegated taste and choice of consumers.

Containing Healthcare Costs by Protecting Nature

Part 1, of this book identified several external factors that may cause our chronic disease state conditions. It is imperative that preventive health experiments be conducted in society in a small-scale manner. The alarming fact is that the destruction of the earth's environment is increasing and not decreasing. Some scientists estimate the extinction rate at 150 species per day. There were an estimated 60 billion hectares of forest on the planet just before World War II. Now, due to logging, cutting firewood, and desertification, there are only 3.6 billion hectares. The World Conservation Union estimates that this forest decline threatens 12.5 percent of the world's 275,000 species of plants and 75 percent of its mammals.[10] The tropical forests of the Amazon contribute to about one third of the world's oxygen and they are disappearing at the rate of 1 percent every year.[11] Yet, we are unsure what the drop in oxygen supply means to our health. Our solutions still seem to be focused at the sub cellular level, when the very cause of sub-cellular damage is external.

The alarming facts on global warming and its relation to our health has already been postulated in earlier chapters. While technological innovations proceed at a rapid pace, we seem to forget their side effects on healthcare. For example, trifluoromethyl sulfur pentafluoride (SF_5CF_3) is 18,000 times more effective as a heat trapper than carbon dioxide, and has an estimated lifespan of 1,000 years. This new greenhouse gas is growing at 6 percent per year. The good news is that it is rare—only .12 parts per trillion in the air. The source of this gas is unknown, but some experts speculate that it may be the breakdown product of a closely related gas used to insulate high voltage equipment.[12]

We not only need to protect the air we breathe, but we also need to preserve our soil against erosion and contamination from several dangerous chemical fertilizers and pesticides that may have deleterious effects on our health. New evidence shows that the most heavily used agricultural chemicals are also hazardous. The herbicide Atrazine, which has been banned in many countries but is still widely used in the U.S., damages the liver, heart, and kidneys. In addition, atrazine, like many synthetic form chemicals, mimics estrogen and has been linked to reproductive disorders, including decreased sperm counts and sterility in males. These chemicals have also been linked to decreased intelligence in both males and females.[13]

Our primary focus on limited issues will not reduce our healthcare costs. We need to look far beyond the state of our world and our interrelationships to truly address our healthcare costs. Unfortunately, our rapid pace of innovation is leaving behind debris that is affecting our health, and we cannot expect the EPA to take care of every single problem. (See Chapter 7 on how we need to address this specific problem).

From a policy perspective, could the U.S. shift its focus from national defense to the environment? We spend more on defense than the next five great military powers put together. We all know that Goliath will always be fought with a sling shot, therefore, it may be well worth our cause to export more technological ideas and solutions on improving the environment, rather than on exporting armaments.

It would be worthy to discuss why the protection of our environment and nature is important for the field of medicine. Now with the Internet and the human genome, many skeptics think the protection of nature is less important and may not even see its connection with medicine.

The invention of synthetic chemistry in the 1930s reduced our reliance in the natural world as the sole source of medicines. Perhaps this may have sent the wrong message on the rampant industrialization of the world at the cost of plundering our natural resources. Mother nature has been devising extraordinary chemicals for more than 3.5 billion years, and new technologies increasingly facilitate our ability to discover, study, manipulate and use these compounds as never before.

For most part, these new technologies have helped us enhance the value of these compounds as a source of healing.

Several promising clues to lifesaving medications of the future are already disappearing from endangered forests, polar ice caps and coral reefs. Ethnobotanist, Mark Plotkin, the author of the well-known book, *Medicine Quest: In Search of Nature's Hidden Cures*, lists scores of superdrugs and miracle pharmaceuticals taken from nature. Tiny cone snails, which live in tropical coral reefs and are described by cancer researchers as "the deadliest creatures on the planet, for their size," have contributed a painkiller more potent than morphine that, unlike morphine, is not addictive. Virus-killing chemicals extracted from a Caribbean sponge led to the discovery of AZT, which halts the progress of AIDS, and some cardiovascular drugs were derived from snake and viper venoms. Five of the world's top 30 drugs are derived from fungi, penicillin being the most notable—one of the least studied and most promising groups of therapeutic organisms. In a Reuters telephone interview, Plotkin mentioned, "I'm sick and tired of hearing people say conservation is a rich man's game, that it's anti-people or anti-business. If you're not concerned about cancer and AIDS and drug resistant bacteria, maybe you shouldn't be interested in conservation. But there are concrete examples of (conservation's) dollar worth and potential."[14]

A study published by Anthony Artuso in *The Journal of Research in Pharmaceutical Economics* once mentioned that in 1993, 79 percent of the top selling 150 pharmaceutical products contained active ingredients that were natural products, derivatives or analogs of natural products.[15] Although it is now recognized that many of nature's plant and animal species are disappearing very rapidly, we can still do something about it, instead of our singular focus being set on rampant industrialization. We have a lot to learn about medicine from animals. Instinct has programmed animals with an inherent knowledge of medicinal plants that our own species is only now beginning to appreciate and study. Monkeys use plants for their medicinal properties, such as to kill parasites. Elephants in Kenya may consume a tree to induce labor and the women of Wa Tongwe in Africa also use this very same plant to induce labor or abortion.[16] This entire field of studying animals use of medicinal plants is called zoopharmacognosy. How humbling that man has to study animals to develop cures for himself. Maybe a solution to develop low-cost medical technologies is to develop a closer link to nature and even better, learn more clearly the source of all instinct. Clearly, animals have better instinct than human beings—dogs know when their masters are about to return home, homing pigeons, even after having traveled thousands of miles, know where they dwell, etc. We may have discovered and unmashed the human genome, but still the basic mysteries on how animals are discovering medicines from the thousands of available plants for specific health conditions is still a mystery to mankind.

From the lowliest maggot (proven to be a great healer), to the giant elephant, to the Shaman in the forest who has a cure for our diabetes, we know we are all connected throughout the world and we all can learn from one another. So, protecting our global environment will only decrease, and not increase our healthcare costs. We need to take less and give more back to nature, lest we become an endangered species ourselves. The very word *physician* is derived from the Greek *physis* meaning "nature," and in this oft-neglected fact is the core of healing's secret.

EMBRACING AN EFFICIENT NATIONAL STRATEGY FOR HEALTHCARE

Physical and biological sciences are two different fields. The strategy in physical sciences has been to question and study matter in order to develop useful inventions for the benefit of society. When physics was stretched to its extreme, people started studying metaphysics, further stretching an objective science to a subjective science. Similarly, in the biological sciences, when people discovered medicine, it was more related to the study of biology, stretched then to the extreme it became a study of the sub-cellular and molecular structures. Stretched to further extremes they became disciplines of the mind, body and spirit. All fields, when stretched to their extremes, blur from objectivity to subjectivity, ultimately leading the scientist, philosopher or saint to come to similar conclusions—the source of creation itself has been the opinion of some of the greatest thinkers and saints. Other than these great and spiritually awakened people, most of us have little clue as to what these things really mean because this is beyond the domain of the intellect. Generally speaking, we are in a comfort zone of objectivity and experiments where a single effect can be correlated to a single cause. Scientific validation of multi-dimensional cause and effect relationships are almost impossible to study in a lab.

Regardless of where science starts and where it ends, one thing is certain, those acts, inventions and innovations, where the intent of the inventor was sincere and was meant to touch the human soul without a commercial motive (as the sole purpose) behind it, truly stood the test of time and were also considered great innovations.

The field of medicine is one field that has numerous examples where the inventor became engrossed in simply finding a cure. Therefore, one should assume that all fields of medicine started with right approach – helping humanity. Scientific validation usually succeeds the right intuition and not vice versa. It is myopic to contest the value of each school of thought as long as the intentions have been right.

While nobody contests the value of several allopathic medications, society could also benefit tremendously from diversity in healthcare. Cultures that have encouraged diversity and variety in every field have progressed. Compare the success of America and its heterogeneous culture and ideas, the mix of races, the opportunities for women and minorities with that of any other nation in the world—we have definitely come a long way. Therefore, even in healthcare this trend is already happening and will continue to happen, it may lower our healthcare costs.

It behooves us to open our arms and embrace all kinds of healthcare technologies that, generally speaking, have honest and admirable motives behind them. When Samuel Hahnemann experimented with medicines on himself, he never cared for his own life. He was considered the father of homeopathy and his philosophy was embraced by Gandhi and Mother Theresa. Homeopathy seems to have several other eminent supporters behind it. Ayurveda, an ancient healthcare system of India, has been practiced for more than 5,000 years. It is a collection of principles of healthy living. In essence, the wisdom is so noble that it is a perfect science on preventive health.

Non-standardization and diversity as a strategy for healthcare will drive costs lower, not higher. We may want to embrace all schools of thoughts of medicine. While freedom of speech has been encouraged in medicine, we also need to encourage freedom of thought, especially when these thoughts have been sincere in helping humanity and have emanated from various cultures. Clayton Christensen of the Harvard School of Business criticizes American healthcare as being a change-averse industry in the United States. According to him, the healthcare industry is trying to preserve outmoded institutions.[17]

Diversification and non-standardization of medicine will complement each of the medical disciplines and will address the severe under-treatment of several diseases, thus benefiting the society and all stakeholders. For example, Ayurveda preaches tongue scraping and has a long essay on its benefits. However, American stores still do not carry tongue scrapers. Only recently, western science addressed haliostasis and the importance of tongue scraping. Ayurveda lists so many other benefits of tongue scraping that people may follow it more seriously. Similarly, there are various other concepts, such as the benefits of fasting, enema, breathing exercises, etc., that are superficial concepts of Ayurveda. The deeper we get into these philosophies, the quicker these concepts may benefit society tremendously. For example, Dr. Andrew Weil, Director of the Program in Integrative Medicine and clinical professor of medicine at the University of Arizona in Tucson, learned some breathing control methods through the study of Yoga. He teaches breathing exercises to all his patients. In his words, "I have seen breath control alone achieve remarkable results: lowering blood pressure, improving long standing patterns of poor digestion, decreasing anxiety and allowing people to get off addictive anti-anxiety drugs, and improving sleep and energy cycles." He further adds, "Not only do these strategies work, something like breathing is a pretty cheap intervention." [18]

The field of Western medicine has complemented the field of herbals or food supplements through the technology of High Performance Liquid Chromatography (HPLC). Without this technology, we would not have known on how to preserve the phyto nutrient content of raw herbs. These are just a few examples on the nature of how all disciplines will eventually become complementary. We have barely scratched the surface in preventive medicine. Preventive medicine is not just about consuming a few herbals from your corner drugstore. Fortunately, there are several new age authors who have opened our eyes on preventive health. Reading each one of their books is a taste of the wisdom that raises our consciousness on preventive health.

While books on preventive health are important, they still do not create a critical mass on preventive health. Therefore, as a national strategy we may want our universities to train different kinds of physicians, homeopaths, ayurvedic practitioners, acupuncturists, practitioners of chinese medicine, tibetan medicine, energetic medicine, etc. Trying to place singular emphasis on allopathic physicians contributes to less diversity in healthcare. Some schools are training allopathic physicians in both eastern and western medicine. This option, while reasonable, still may not lower our healthcare costs.

Let me provide an analogy: would one enter a restaurant that serves chinese, mexican, american, and italian food or would one prefer instead a food court where one can walk to separate and distinct restaurant booths to pick the right choice of a food. The former strategy will increase the cost of the food, whereas the latter will decrease the cost because of focus and efficiencies in specialization. Similarly, even in healthcare when we train allopathic physicians to be proficient in all schools of medicine our costs will not decrease they will only increase—just as a restaurant (specializing in all foods) strategy vs. a food court (like the ones in a mall) strategy. When allopathic physicians get trained in all medical disciplines (eastern and western), power will be in the hands of a select few which could result in monopolies on medical treatment. For this reason, such training should not be a national strategy. In fact, lower cost disciplines may become more expensive due to the simple nature of market economics.

Instead, we need to broaden our options by training different kinds of practitioners of medicine. Our country may need to have a food court that fosters a philosophy of medicine that caters to all tastes and beliefs. This is certainly one method where we could address the severe under-treatment of disease in several classes while raising the level of preventive health nationwide. Having practitioners in different fields of medicine provides a true meaning to diversity and encourages all fields of medicine to eventually become truly complementary while providing choice to the consumer at an affordable cost.

The only country to my knowledge that embraced all forms of healthcare disciplines similar to that of a food court strategy is India. India has practitioners ranging from Tibetan medicine to the most advanced cardiac surgeons. The system allows the poor, the rich, and consumers with different beliefs and tastes to choose and follow whatever medicine best suits their mind, body and spirit temperament. It is surprising that all forms thrive equally well with minimal controversy. In every city you can find practitioners of all different kinds of medicine. By any means, I am not trying to justify the healthcare system of India, because it has several structural defects. In addition, population and poverty have distorted the healthcare system of India. However, the point I am trying to make is that the government of India adopted an open-minded attitude towards medicine. Although Ayurveda was born in India, the government never let the system become totally entrenched with this form. They opened their doors to western medicine, homeopathy, reiki, etc. Germany is another good example where they have a Commission E, a government body that approves the use of herbals. Homeopathy is also popular in Germany, since it is the country from where it originated. India itself may have about 100,000 practitioners in homeopathy. Countries like China have adopted a system that is predominately based on herbal remedies. Herbal remedies account for up to half of their total medicinal consumption.

The stated national strategy does not imply that traditional healthcare companies must start embracing different schools of thought or technologies, rather it says that these companies should participate in this competitive process. Traditional companies should try to keep improving on their existing technologies, make it better, safer, and more useful for the society and the environment. Rather than jumping from point A to point B, they may want to follow a sequential path of innovation with a non-linear approach to the thinking process. They should ultimately make their technologies affordable and if possible have the patient manage their own health with little interference.

For example, before the 1980s most patients with diabetes used an inaccurate urine test to measure their glucose levels, or visited a doctor who drew a blood sample and then measured its glucose content on an expensive piece of laboratory equipment. Today, patients pack miniature blood glucose meters with them wherever they go. They mange most aspects of the disease that previously required much more professional involvement. They get far higher quality of care more conveniently and at a lower cost. Similarly, people with coronary artery disease are now treated in a lower cost setting. When care was complex in the past, people refused treatment. It is exactly because of this that we need diversity in healthcare. The more affordable technologies become, the fewer problems of under-treatment. Once this is better addressed, our expenses may decrease. Another example is that of a flu vaccine. Belgian researchers are working on a vaccine that would need be given only once in a lifetime, rather than every year. While improvements in product are necessary for lowering costs, innovations in the methods of appropriate treatment strategy are equally important. For example, researchers now believe that giving antibiotics at higher doses for shorter periods of time makes it more difficult for the bacteria to become resistant. This stratagem was effective in treating the common ear infection known as *otitis media.* A course of antibiotics no longer than three days—and, in some cases, just a single shot—was enough to cure the infection. Another example is a five-day course of azithromycin, rather than 10 days of penicillin, to clear up a sore throat due to *streptococcus A* infection. A shorter course of antibiotics using the right one in the higher dose for a lesser period of time not only may be as effective as the traditional treatment but also is cheaper and is likely to have fewer side effects.[19] Another example of a treatment strategy that would save costs is with respect to the elderly sometimes taking more medications than may be necessary. Jerry Avorn, a researcher at Brigham and Women's Hospital in Boston, says systematically reviewing patients' medications "may be one of the most important medical interventions you can do."[20]

Every company will have a niche, every company will have a place, and every consumer will be satisfied if we set our vision high and aim to reduce the costs of healthcare through continuous and improved product, process, and strategy innovations by being focused on a defined path.

This stated strategy on each healthcare philosophy staying on its stated path could be threatened if we allow ourselves to interfere with the inherent innovative processes of each of these schools of thought. For example, if we allow ourselves to re-import the several allopathic medications invented in this country, then we could make medicine less cost effective in the long run. Trying to find low-cost solutions to higher-cost alternatives may also disappear. Trying to find cures that vastly impoverish the world may be out of reach for several companies. For example, in the sub-Saharan Africa, AIDS and malaria limit the life expectancy to only 40 years.[21] About 2 million people in Africa die each year because of malaria.[22] Neither conventional nor non-conventional forms of medicine have found a complete cure for these epidemics. However, if each philosophy stayed on its path without interference, we may someday find a cure. Ignoring these epidemics may only increase impoverishment in the world with further devastating consequences across the world. Such reform initiatives like the re-importation of medicine are the adverse side effects of not developing an attitude for diversity in healthcare.

It is also important that each culture and each philosophy remain on its stated path (while complementing as appropriate their core philosophies). No single culture or no single system will have all of the answers for all of the variegated kinds of disease conditions. The best strategy is for different cultures and schools of thought to learn from each other without belittling the concepts and philosophies of each. The great anthropologist Weston La Barre, who collaborated with R.E. Schultes on his early peyote research, wrote of the South American Indian:

As scientists we can not afford the luxury of an ethnocentric snobbery which assumes *a priori* that primitive cultures have nothing whatsoever to contribute to civilization. Our civilization is, in fact, a compendium of such borrowings, and it is demonstrable error to believe that contacts of "higher" and "lower" cultures show benefits flowing exclusively in one direction. Indeed, a good case could probably be made that in the long run it is the "higher" culture which benefits the more through being enriched, while the "lower" culture not uncommonly disappears entirely as a result of the contact.[23]

The following practical example shows how a lower culture could have benefited a higher culture. While watching a TV report on sea otters soaked up by the 1989 *Exxon Valdez* oil spill, an Alabama hairdresser noticed that otter fur soaked up oil extremely well. The hair dresser replicated the phenomena he saw on the television by sweeping the hair from the salon floor, stuffed it into a pair of tights to make a dummy otter, and threw it into a baby pool filled with water and a gallon of motor oil. In two minutes, he reported, "the water was crystal clear." Salon clients who worked for NASA put him in touch with an expert there who ran a large-scale test. It found that "1.4 million pounds of hair contained in mesh pillows could have soaked up the entire *Exxon Valdez* oil spill in a week," saving much of the $2 billion Exxon spent to capture only 12 percent of the 11 million gallons spilled.[24] The irony is that a hair dresser came up with a better idea than even the most brilliant scientists at *Exxon*. This is a clear example of how a lower culture could have benefited a higher culture. It also demonstrates the need for diversity and non-standardization in healthcare with respect to embracing different ideas, philosophies, etc.

ALLOCATING RESOURCES FOR THE EFFICIENT IMPLEMENTATION OF STRATEGIES

The previous section detailed the rationale for embracing an efficient healthcare strategy that would work to lower costs. Allocation of national resources and policy strategy often go together. The schematic diagram below may help the reader understand the current allocation of our resources.

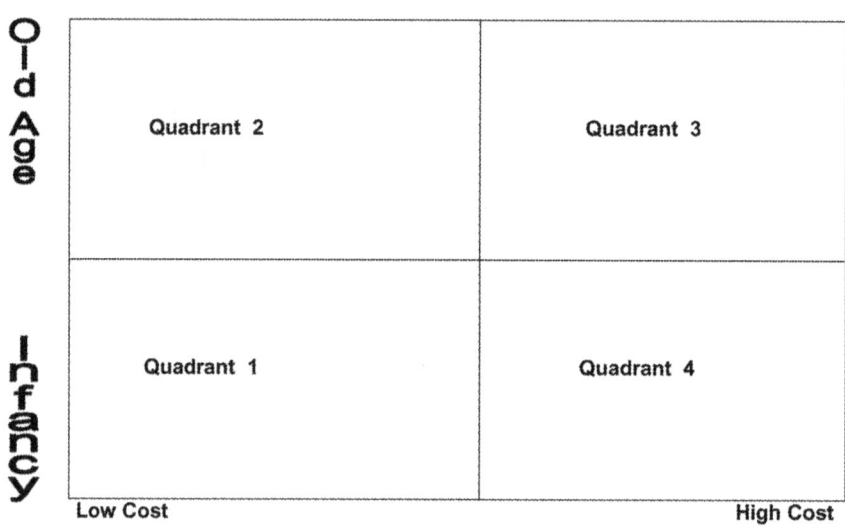

Healthcare Technologies

On the X axis is the range of all healthcare technologies from the lowest to the highest cost. On the Y axis is the average time span of a human life, ranging say from 0 to 80 years. As people age, the costs of healthcare also seem to increase. This schematic helps us assess the current allocation of our national resources. The general perception is that our resources and our energy are concentrated in Quadrant 3. The more we focus our resources on Quadrant 3, the higher the increases in cost. When our resources gradually shift from Quadrant 3 to Quadrant 2, and Quadrant 4 to Quadrant 1, we can anticipate an overall decrease in cost. Clayton Christensen of the Harvard School of Business would probably have deemed the technologies in quadrant 1 and 2 as being, "disruptive technologies" since they threaten established business models. I would like to call them "socially responsible technologies". From a practical point of view, our resources and innovations may be allocated in any quadrant, but eventually they need to shift to quadrants 1 or 2 based on the demographics of the market. Some innovations will always remain in Quadrant 3. These are the exceptions. As a society, we have a responsibility to support complex medical problems. Some interventions will be costly and some interventions will have cheaper alternatives. Finally, our role as scientists and responsible citizens is to find the right balance.

When we observe the healthcare costs of the U.S. versus that of other countries, we realize that we have leaned more heavily on quadrant 3 than other quadrants. The pace continues to accelerate even in our research endeavors. For example, many biologists, chemists, and physicians in this country are trying to unlock the secrets of aging. Most of these scientists imagine that aging will be slowed by taking a pill or by surgery such as gene or stem cell therapy. Controversy rages over all these techniques. Some are being outlawed, and all are hotly debated. The Food and Drug Administration (FDA) will not approve a drug given solely to prevent or slow aging because the FDA does not classify aging as a disease. On the contrary, if these scientists shifted their resources into quadrant 1 technologies, they may be forced to consider reaching the same end-goal through low cost interventions such as "breath-control," since this has had demonstrated positive effects on the mind. It is the mind that rules the body. The best built computer is worthless if it has a faulty operating system. All of these issues are highly complex, controversial, and even debatable. However, the law of supply and demand will eventually drive the market towards quadrants 1 and 2. This will happen only if we open our doors to market forces, diversity, and cultural openness. Consumers, organizations, researchers, and physicians will all benefit if they use quadrant 1 and 2 as a springboard for all their ideas with respect to developing products or services. These institutions will also benefit by shifting their existing technologies from quadrant 3&4 to 1&2.

In real life, however, the relentless pursuit of growth and the current healthcare infrastructure leave existing technologies in quadrants 3&4 unable to shift to quadrant 1&2. Paradoxically, the focus shifts to creating further new innovations in the same quadrant 3&4. Unfortunately, our current system does not provide incentives for companies or people to shift from quadrant 3&4 to 1&2 (see Chapter 5). For example, in his book, *Competition and Monopoly in Medical care*, H.E. Frech points out that the more insurance coverage an enrollee has, the less willing he or she is to search for lower prices. The worst type of insurance, in Frech's opinion, is the kind that provides 100 percent coverage (like Medicaid and much of Medicare) which generates no incentive for the consumer to shop around. He argues that this consumer complacency cedes enormous power to physicians and insurers at the expense of patients.[25] This is an example of one kind of market force where the consumer complacency does not drive institutions to shift to lower cost quadrants. However, in a scenario where consumers are free to opt-out of their employer-sponsored plans and purchase healthcare coverage with before-tax income, they will go in search of the insurance product that best suits their individual needs. This infusion of flexibility, choice and cash is a type of market force that may compel several parties to gradually shift from higher cost to lower cost quadrants.

As long as several of the market imperfections continue to occur, we may not see a decline in the overall costs of healthcare, unless of course, market forces change the paradigm. Also, more innovations are needed in quadrant 1 (Chapters 1 and 2, have already offered some key original ideas and innovations). Some healthcare technologies like vaccines quickly shifted from Quadrant 3 to Quadrant 1. This experiment thus saved the lives of millions of children all over the world. Similarly, technologies that displaced surgeries can be considered of making a shift from a higher cost to the lower cost quadrants.

The next section is a comparison on the growth of the computer industry versus the healthcare industry. It demonstrates how the computer industry quickly shifted from quadrants 3&4 to 1&2 from a cost perspective. This shift was associated with increased growth at a lower unit cost. Society had a better perception of value with increased growth because there was greater quality at a lower unit cost. Therefore, in the long run, even in healthcare creation of value can only be achieved by producing greater quality at a lower unit cost.

GROWTH OF THE COMPUTER INDUSTRY VS. THE GROWTH OF THE HEALTHCARE INDUSTRY

In 1999, the internet economy generated revenue in excess of half a trillion dollars (roughly half of what we spend on healthcare) and added 650,000 jobs. The internet workforce now surpasses the entire active U.S. military, insurance, communication, and public utilities industries. It is twice the size of the airline, chemical and allied products, legal, and real estate industries.[26] A retail computer salesperson once mentioned to me that on average a person would spend about $15,000 on technology-related products and services in his lifetime. I wondered if these purchases would match or exceed healthcare costs on a per person basis in the coming years. Immediately it struck me then on why people are not concerned with major investments in computer products vs. investments in healthcare. These are some hypotheses:

1. Differences in demographics.

2. Growth with diversity is true growth, ultimately lowering costs.

3. Although the computer industry continues to grow, presumably much faster than the healthcare industry, a consumer knows and understands that costs are becoming more affordable. Therefore, he is not concerned, even if the overall industry continues to grow. On a personal level he has found a sense of satisfaction with zero assistance from an outside financier.

4. People who purchase computers and related services, including corporations, perceive a technological purchase as an investment

into the future. However, it is questionable whether we (including payers) consider the purchase of health as an investment or as an expense. If it is the latter, we should go deep into ourselves and find out all of the reasons.

5. Perception of value in a technological purchase is immediate, more tangible, and is almost considered as an essential need in the present day. Healthcare, however, is a subjective and an individual experience.

    Comparisons between the computer industry and the healthcare industry should offer us some clues on low cost approaches, diversity and choice. Growth may sometimes lower costs and not increase them. Overall growth in the right manner may change perceptions of people and their spending patterns.

CONCLUSION

A desired strategy for healthcare must be to provide diversity, non-standardization, affordability, and an approach to making medicine more affordable. This can be accomplished by seeking out simple solutions to complex and intractable problems by providing a plethora of choices that satisfy every single customer—rich or poor, conventional or non-conventional belief systems. Such an approach will lower costs and raise the overall consciousness on preventive health. Diversity is complementary and not displacing, diversity retains independence, establishes symbiosis, and provides general well being for all consumers of healthcare. It provides growth opportunities for a variety of industries, expands markets, and reduces the cumulative costs of healthcare. In such systems, individuals and corporations gravitate towards the most efficient forms of healthcare that appeal to their intuition, imagination and reasoning. To some extent, this has been demonstrated above on how it happened in the computer industry.

In the long run, only diversity in healthcare will address the chronic under-treatment of several disease classes and therefore protect the long-term health of the nation. Finally, our approach to healthcare must be humble, environmental, and open-minded to all philosophies and cultures. We should foster the growth of each single philosophy rather than claim dominance of any single philosophy or school of thought.

4

Some Innovations in Information Technology That will Lower Healthcare Costs

L et us now transition to see how innovations in Informational Technology could change the healthcare landscape regardless of how the Government fosters change. Interspersed within the essay are both existing and theoretical innovations.

Advancements in Informational Technology devices and software will shift healthcare from a centralized structure to a decentralized structure. This does not mean that product branding and marketing would disappear, it only implies that highly-informed decisions would be made on an increasingly microcosmic level. Companies, therefore, may want to position themselves in order to conform to this paradigm. Healthcare has and always will be an information-intensive service industry. The ability to measure outcomes and improve performance—the process of innovation—and to share such information rapidly is at the heart of the democratization of medicine and the catalyst for patient-centered care. Most new medical knowledge pertains to methods to prevent or treat disease with greater success, involving less time, money, and pain. And these methods change so rapidly that, as Donald Lindberg, director of the National Library of Medicine has noted, "If a young conscientious physician was determined to keep up with medical advances by reading two articles from a peer-reviewed journal every day, by the end of one year he or she would have fallen behind 800 years in medical reading."[1] A German economist and policy expert, Wilfred Prewo, has astutely framed this issue when he observed that healthcare systems, like all other economic sectors, are moving from the "machine age" into the "information age."[2]

However, with technology, diverse information from several different places will be segmented, organized, and disseminated in a fashion that an end-user will be able to easily utilize. At the present time, healthcare information is extremely fragmented. More than 70 million consumers are using the Internet to search for health information. Their biggest hurdles are finding common ground or sifting through a variety of different sources on a similar subject.[3] Slowly and eventually all this may change. Patients will be put at the epicenter of the healthcare system.

E-technologies are making steady gains in empowering both physicians and consumers and are transforming the way they think. This may have tremendous implications for the healthcare industry. These forces will make the industry efficient and fortunately lower our healthcare costs. These technologies will provide equal power in different ways to both the physician and consumer. In a matter of seconds, people will be able to navigate and access the best data organized in a fashion that an end-user can understand. Complexity will emerge due to the plethora of gadgets that will be available. Through time, however, only the true winners will be left standing.

PORTABLE TECHNOLOGIES THAT MAY LOWER HEALTHCARE COSTS

For most physicians, medicine has become too complex to practice from a dog-eared textbook. If a physician were to practice true "evidence-based" medicine, he or she would have to skim through thousands of articles a year to snare clinically useful findings. Medical practice has never been the scientific endeavor we imagine. Studies have shown that doctors pay less attention to research findings than to colleagues and drug-company representatives.[4]

However, a slew of products—from wireless, palm-sized PCs to scanners, speech recognition recorders, and Internet-based software programs—are going change the way physicians access information. At Michigan State University and the University of Virginia, some 200 physicians are road-testing the first palm top version of InfoRetriever (IR). IR is an information-rich device that is tightly focused on patient care. With IR, you punch in 'migraine' and you get a summary of a clinical research related to migraines.

This is what Dr. Renier Brentjens, an internist and oncology fellow at New York's Sloan Kettering Hospital has to say about hand-held PCs: "The possibilities are endless; You can take notes, get a pharmacy drug listing, or input and reference cancer stages, chemotherapy schedules, and drug dosages anywhere, anytime, at your fingertips." Another plus, he adds, is easy access to a patient's database: "If I get called and don't have a chart, especially in the middle of the night, I can check up on things like allergies and drug interactions that I wouldn't have necessarily memorized."[5]

There are now several similar devices on the market. For example, the Compaq iPAQ can store up to 1,000 medications and formularies. All of these gizmos and gadgets may soon flood the market. There are several examples of how doctors are saving their insurers thousands of dollars through use of these gadgets.

Once HMOs have figured out how doctors use these gadgets or have documented savings for the HMO, they will begin to offer more training to doctors on the use of these technologies. At the moment, only one in four physicians' uses a computer at work.[6] With training from managed care companies and new young doctors entering the workforce, this paradigm is going to change. Portable databases will make doctors more efficient and help them practice better medicine. This, in my opinion, will be the <u>first stage</u> of the portable revolution. HMOs will probably conduct studies to verify per member-per month costs on those who use these devices versus those who do not use these devices. If the benefits are superior on the use of these devices, we will see a proliferation in training.

I predict the <u>second stage</u> of the portable database revolution to be focused on the consumer rather than the physician. This revolution has already started on the Internet, and with the growth of on-line pharmacies such as PlanetRx and Drugstore.com, people now have the option to sift through the information explosion on both alternative and conventional forms of medicine. However, as consumers begin to bear more of the burden of healthcare costs, they will lean more towards the use of portable databases. The second stage of the portable database revolution will be in alternative medicine, where a consumer will be able to figure out what philosophy best suits him or her. The second stage will proceed in a slow and arduous manner. Consumers will still rely on their doctors but will lean towards these technologies when they have exhausted their conventional options, or are forced to pay more out-of-pocket costs for healthcare. If healthcare payers transition to a defined benefit plan, the second stage of the portable revolution is likely to accelerate.

The <u>third stage</u> of the portable database revolution will be in integrated medicine. Databases will merge and combine the best modalities of treatment in both conventional and non-conventional forms of medicine. All this will take time. Perhaps between the years 2010 and 2020 we will see an explosion in information and gadgets that we have never seen before. Smart companies will embrace and adapt their vision to grow with these technologies.

Somewhere between the second and third stages, the gene therapy revolution may be incorporated into these portable databases. The gene-based technologies can do great good, and depending on the nature of the technology, can also result in great harm. In large measure, the issues being confronted for gene-based technologies could be the same ones that will be faced whenever a powerful new technology is developed. Ethics, safety, and debate must be focused to keep the cost of these technologies in balance.

IMPLICATIONS FOR INDUSTRY AND GOVERNMENT

The Government may want to be open to these new technologies also, and implement them while it reshapes healthcare. Policies that interfere with democratic entrepreneurship may put several industries out of balance and may contribute to a lopsided growth in the economy. Entrepreneurial spirit must be encouraged. This approach enlightens the public, increases their education, and provides them choice to make more intelligent decisions.

Industry will have to closely observe the implications of several new technologies, including Information Technology. The important thing is that a surfeit of these new devices in information technology and organization of data on healthcare will not diminish the opportunities for companies to market or sell their products. On the contrary, it will increase opportunities to sell more effectively to an informed customer by an informed sales representative. Therefore, companies may want to embrace and shape their systems, strategies, and infrastructure so that they ultimately become contributors to a reduction in overall healthcare costs. Companies who successfully participate in this process will survive and prosper.

All of these technologies may also give rise to a new breed of entrepreneurs, as well as several new professions. Physician offices may create new positions where people become experts on several different portable databases. New businesses will emerge that will match patient profiles to portable database technology. The role of drug representatives could also change from pure product sales to those who will synthesize a variety of information for the physician. They could potentially play a secondary "techno-role" that a physician would not have time to assume. Genomics may also change the representative's role. Instead of merchandising one or two drugs, they will now develop treatment portfolios for the physicians' patient mix. A lot of companies may experience diminishing impact of their centralized marketing strategies relative to their historic position. A decentralized and a creative way of managing a business in the physicians' office through the marketing of several connected products and services may become more fashionable.

Healthcare companies will survive in this game through several partnerships amongst several different kinds of industry. Global e-charity and consolidation of websites (an innovative concept described below), as well as several other factors will raise awareness for healthcare all across the globe. This awareness will offer several potential opportunities for healthcare firms. Companies will survive by adapting themselves to localized strategies. Strategy shifts will take place to manage complex processes. It is hard to surmise how individual companies will transform themselves, but transformation of healthcare on a macro and a micro-level are imminent in the long run.

Ultimately, partnerships with both for-profit and non-profit companies in totally different industries and concepts that truly benefit the consumer and touch their hearts will succeed. With the growth in the information explosion, the synthesis of complex information will make all parties and customer groups equally powerful. The challenge of the industry will be to address these different groups of customers in a cost-efficient manner. The secret for the industry will be to combine concepts of social entrepreneurship with for-profit concepts. Simple and centralized approaches to linear sales growth may tend to produce lower returns.

CONSOLIDATING WEBSITES

The healthcare industry is certainly in need of some air traffic control on the Internet. Right now, it appears that different websites seem to crash into each other and cause confusion to the consumers. Prestigious non-profit institutions could take leadership in consolidating different websites. For example, the American Lung Association could consolidate several different websites on lung-related diseases by assimilating knowledge on all different areas. These websites could take clues on the example of a consumer wanting to research a company before he/she invests money in the stock of a particular company. Nowadays, even a high school or young college student knows how to research and invest in a company by going on the Internet. The information is easy to navigate. Healthcare information should be organized in a similar manner. Investment in a company makes us navigate through similar patterns of thought process. Although two completely divergent decisions, the logical process flow may have some similarities.

INNOVATIONS IN SOFTWARE THAT WILL ALLOW PEOPLE TO PREDICT THEIR LONGEVITY

In this section, I recommend corporations develop a software that can predict an individual's longevity. The goal of this software must be to offer an individual a preventive health model that he or she can easily pursue.

Bill Sharpe, a Professor of Economics at the University of Washington and a winner of the 1990 Nobel Prize in Economics co-founded Financial Engines to bring undiluted modern portfolio theory to the masses. In late 1998, the firm began rolling out user-friendly, Internet-based software that gives 401(k) plan participants the same sophisticated forecasting and asset—allocation tools that are used by pension-fund managers. Today Financial Engines provides its advisory service to 550 organizations and 1.7 million retirement plan participants.[7] Financial Engines doesn't promise a definitive yes or no answer to the all important question of whether an investment will have enough money at retirement. Instead, it uses simulation analysis to come up the probability that an investment goal can be reached and then provides advice on improving the odds.

Similarly, when an individuals' electronic medical records are tied to a similar software such as the Financial Engines, an individual can forecast the quality of his health status based on his commitment to a certain set of lifestyle modifications and/or compliance with medications, etc. Such innovations in software may reinforce the value of better preventive health and may help lower healthcare costs.

GLOBALIZING HEALTH CHARITY TO LOWER HEALTHCARE COSTS

The end of the twentieth century will perhaps be remembered as the age of the Internet. It inspired and fostered young talent, sped up the velocity of capital, attacked cost, inspired new ideas, lowered price, allowed the stock market to work smarter and faster, suppressed inflation, and created a few millionaires out of the plethora of start-up technology companies. One thing, however, fell by the wayside: an opportunity to tap the potential of Internet to globalize charitable healthcare and reduce healthcare costs.

The new millennium can now focus on creating social entrepreneurs who can carry the mantle of creating several start-up e-charity companies individualized for serving healthcare needs of several nations. The concepts that went into concocting "for-profit" Internet businesses can now be easily applied to charitable causes and reduce overall healthcare costs across the globe.

The benefits of the application of e-commerce to charity are immense and immediate. It will allow a charitable donor to take pride in knowing how and where his charity benefited humanity. Bound together by a digital mesh, this idea can allow all the countries of the world, including our own, to minimize disparities in the wealth and knowledge of healthcare. Individuals and organizations will be empowered by the concept to erase the boundaries of the world. This is how this idea would work:

Social entrepreneurs could establish a site similar to eBay. Hospitals and individuals all across the globe would access this site to list their donations, such as used diagnostic equipment, used medical books, computers, medical CDs, used electronic components, used medical devices, eye glasses, hearing aids, prosthetics, etc., on the e-charity website. Hospitals all across the world and the U.S. would access the site and order the listed items for a reasonable charge, or the donor can offer it for free. Health charities such as 'Gift of Sight,' would have hyperlinks built into these websites

More fortunate institutions and individuals would be connected directly with the less fortunate American or foreign institutions and individuals. The lack of a middleman in the process may provide efficiencies in supply-chain warehousing, distribution, etc. Such a system offers efficiencies of time, cost, and manpower.

Unlike the U.S., for the developing world this would be a giant leap because an e-charity company specializing in healthcare could simply circumvent the poor infrastructure of these countries. The concept allows delivery of goods to the doorstep of a hospital, charitable institution, or an individual recipient with minimal infrastructure obstacles, a major deterrent for charity across the globe. Various intermediaries and middlemen in these countries also compound the problems. According to Jeff Skoll, Vice President of eBay, intermediaries will find themselves "disintermediated" in eBay. Disintermediation is the single biggest advantage for an e-Charity company.[8]

An e-charity company specializing in satisfying healthcare needs creates efficiencies on a global basis through the elimination of waste in society. Like other charitable institutions, an e-charity company would provide tax-deductible benefits to the charitable donor. As the world globalizes, charity becomes a two-way street, the U.S. will not only be the giver, but also the receiver of the fruits of charity due to global advancement of knowledge and commerce. For example, when major diagnostic equipment fails in a hospital in the U.S., it could access a spare part sometimes free of charge from a different country by accessing the website.

The 1998 United Nations Human Development Report states that even though global economic output has increased sixfold since 1950, 3 billion people, more than half the world's population, live on less than $2 per day. Global advancement in knowledge and commerce can only come through embracing equity on a worldwide basis.[9] The report also notes that in 1960 the income of 20 percent of the world's people who lived in the richest countries was 30 times the income of the 20 percent who lived in the poorest countries.[10] By 1995 the ratio was 82 to one. Using Congressional Budget Office data, the Center on Budget and Policy Priorities conclude that from 1977 to 1994, the after-tax income of the richest one percent of U.S. households increased by 72 percent, while that of the bottom 20 percent fell 16 percent.[11] E-Charity is just one avenue that can easily touch healthcare and create equity without cash donations. It is said that democracies that trade with one another almost never go to war. If true, e-Charity companies specializing in healthcare could become the harbingers for world peace since they would symbolize an electronic version of a World Health (Care) Organization formed by local citizens and the hospitals of the world.

In an e-charity company, an individual should be allowed to ship the materials on his own to an end user almost anywhere. It is possible for an e-Charity company to reimburse shipping costs based on broad guidelines for specific items. An e-Charity company would raise money through advertisements, a yearly subscription fee, etc. Administration could be easily managed on the website without any person or party leaving home.

The idea and the logistics for establishing such a site are simple and inexpensive; it is the leadership and social entrepreneurship that will have to come from "not-for-profit" entrepreneurs in the healthcare field.

The e-Charity site also has the potential to extend the charity of medical services or serve as a clearing-house for exchange programs. This concept would accelerate high-cost technologies to borrow ideas from lower cost technologies, conversely, lower cost technologies could borrow ideas from higher cost technologies to optimize on further efficiencies. For example, an exchange program between universities, where a renowned acupuncturist from China could visit the U.S. and a renowned Cardiac surgeon from the U.S. could visit China. Such exchange programs even in the fields of medical research may help contain our costs. All of these concepts were covered in theory in Chapter 3.

PART III

5

Innovations in Policy and Reform that may Lower Healthcare Costs

S ociety has brought to fore the various innovative ideas that are more focused on reform and policy. These issues and innovations are centered on the general health and well being of society. Surprisingly, these issues that touch our hearts and minds also may have the indirect benefit of lowering our healthcare costs. However, these issues should not be looked at from the point of view of lowering our healthcare costs. That should not be our goal. On the contrary, they should be looked at from a quality-of-life perspective. At times, quality-of-life issues may raise healthcare costs, but at other times these issues may lower healthcare costs. This is what healthcare is all about.

Let us start with some examples. As a society we refrain from debating issues that are considered taboo, such as death and dying. The most challenging reform is to motivate patients advocate for a dignified or more comfortable death. This may increase the quality of life for the patient and it may or may not lower healthcare costs, however, on balance the right approach always works towards optimizing costs.

Dr. Ira Byock, author of *Dying Well: Peace and Possibilities at the End of Life,* believes that the baby boomers, who demanded many of the changes in the way we came into the world, will be equally insistent on changing the way we live. Studies show that nearly half of Americans die in pain.[1] According to Dr. Byock, the debate over dying in

America has focused on a narrow question: Is there a right to die? But that struggle, so agonizing, so dramatic, overshadows practical questions that will prove more important for us: How will we die, and can we die more comfortably?[2]

Some people who die in pain want Jack Kevorkian as an alternative. As a society, we should not hide the issue of death, it should be open for debate. If you want physician-assisted suicide, you'll need to move to Oregon, the only state in which doctors may legally administer a lethal dose of medication. Some other states like Hawaii are considering it. Only one third of Oregon residents die in institutions, in contrast to the 75 percent national average.[3] As a state, Oregon spends the lowest amount of money on inpatient care in the final six months of life.[4] The issue of death is a highly complex and a debatable issue. If States encourage physician-assisted suicide solely to lower costs then the ethics of these methods are questionable because death is such a complex issue. In my opinion, it should be left to the choice of the individual. Death like birth should be as natural as possible. If someone were to prolong my death by using high-tech gadgets that cause more pain and anguish, and a financial burden to both immediate family and society, I would prefer to die. Similarly, I would not prefer suicide due to religious beliefs. As one can see here, death has several moral, religious, ethical, and highly complex and charged implications.

Several well-intentioned initiatives have already started in this area. For example, the Patient Self –Determination Act , which took effect in 1991, stipulates that hospitals seek advance directives or living wills from patients. Advance Directives are intended to clarify whether a patient prefers to desire more aggressive treatment. Also, in an effort hailed as a major step in improving care for the dying, 14 medical associations and the Joint Commission on Accreditation of Healthcare Organizations have signed on to a set of core principles for end-of-life care.[5] Most hospitals prefer living wills or advance directives. Unfortunately, because these subjects are taboo nothing is accomplished. The least we could do is have the government offer a $1,000 one time tax exemption for people who prepare living wills and/or advance directives, this lays the onus of the ethics on the concerned individual and hopefully will cause less anguish in several families and will address to lower costs in the right manner. Correct ethics will ultimately lower costs or optimize costs and not increase costs.

The other reform issue we need to challenge is the use of cellular phones in cars. There is an intensive debate going on in several states that cell phones are distractive during driving and thus are one reason for several accidents. Intuitively this makes sense, however, as a society we want proof till we may have some verifiable deaths—as though life was just a commodity. In 1997, *The New England Journal of Medicine* reported that motorists who use cell phones are four times more likely to crash, and equated their use with drunk driving.[6] In a three-year study of Oklahoma crash data, researchers linked cell phone use with a ninefold increase in fatalities. According to the National Highway Traffic Safety Administration (NHTSA), Oklahoma is the only state to have such data. The political clout of 76 million cell phone users often dwarfs the implementation of strong measures. Yes, cell phones are useful during emergencies, however, they could also be used for conversations in service or rest areas. Cars are not meant to be places to conduct business or have social conversations. These are important reform issues that may save billions of dollars in healthcare costs, not to mention the agony and the suffering that could be avoided by millions of families.

Most people are already familiar with the tobacco industry and the ill effects of smoking. The irony and the paradox is that the Government subsidizes the tobacco industry, and yet also spends billions of dollars on fighting this industry. We may need to determine our priorities as a society.

Issues like medical malpractice awards, the limitless amount of monetary damages that our society allows us to claim, etc., have caused several imperfections in our healthcare system and have increased our healthcare costs. While these issues can increase the quality of our lives, they also can increase costs when abused to the extreme. When we can sue for limitless amounts of damages, our behavior changes accordingly; we are less likely to actively participate in reform until we realize a serious consequence. For example, the European society takes a more active role in the introduction of certain bioengineered foods than their American counterparts. This does not imply that if we lower the amount one can be awarded in a lawsuit that we are trying to condone the introduction of any specific technology or service, or is trying to absolve an industry of its responsibility to society. It just means that we need to place both industry and society on an equal footing regarding a variety of issues that involve the general health and well being of society. Trying to achieve an optimal balance on the amount that can be awarded in a lawsuit makes all parties more, and not less, involved.

There are several issues of reform where we need to be innovative, not to reduce or lower costs, but increase our quality of life. A reform issue that has almost been unchallenged is on achieving a Medical School Degree.

MEDICAL SCHOOL DEGREE

Almost all of the Universities in the United States will admit students to a medical school after completion of a four-year undergraduate degree, regardless of their field of specialization, provided they pass their MCATs (Medical College Admission Test). It is difficult to comprehend the rationale for this policy, but surprisingly this policy has not been challenged or even questioned.

If the rationale for making a medical degree program into a cumulative eight-year program, (four year undergraduate degree plus another four years of medical school), was to limit the supply of physicians, then this rationale has proven incorrect. We need to understand the basis of why a medical degree program is an eight-year program. If the intent was to restrict supply this could have been achieved by imposing selection criteria based on an aptitude test for medical school. If the basis for medical school admittance was to understand human responsibility gained through an extended period of study, then pharmacists have as much responsibility for human lives as physicians. We live in an age where there are a plethora of medicines, yet pharmacists achieve their degree after high school. Looking at the issue from all angles, the idea that medicine requires a four-year undergraduate degree as a prerequisite is hard to understand. Therefore, medicine like pharmacy should be a six-year program after high school.

In Britain, the Government pays all tuition throughout a students undergraduate degree, this includes even obtaining a medical degree. In the U.S., the system pays for our education until high school. In some ways, we compensate for this since our healthcare system, unlike Britain, is not nationalized. The Federal Government in the U.S. however, subsidizes the training of resident physicians in amounts that are expected to approach $7.5 billion for the year 2000.[7] There is debate on drastically lowering these subsidies. Should this occur, residents in the U.S. may get reduced stipends than what they may currently be receiving.

Younger students (elementary, middle, and high) appear more compassionate and open-minded than many adults or even students in a four-year undergraduate degree program. Their ideals for voluntary work, a sincere interest to help humanity, appear more genuine. In the words of Dr. Sherwin B. Nuland, "Medical school admission committees look for winners: the highest GPAs, the highest scores on Medical College Admissions Test, the most glowing reports about undergraduate achievements. They like to see stratospheric numbers and florid adjectives. In view of this emphasis, it is a wonder that they manage to admit as many idealistic young people to the profession as they do."[8] Surveys of medical school applicants demonstrate the different motives that encourage men and women who enter the medical profession "Ask men why they're entering medicine, and they say 'prestige and salary.' Ask women why they are entering medicine, and they say 'helping people'."[9] It would be interesting to research the backgrounds of physicians who belong to the organization *Doctors Without Borders*. I surmise that it was not their GPA's or glowing academic records that won them the Nobel Peace Prize, rather it was the altruistic and idealistic nature that these doctors exhibited.

If we really want these idealistic young people to obtain a medical school degree, let us then provide them an opportunity to obtain their degree after high school education. Human beings are a product of mind, body and spirit. A doctor needs to treat all of these. They must assume to be responsible for the totality of a patients life. It is questionable that this talent is somehow gained through a four-year undergraduate course of study.

In some countries, people do become doctors after a four, five, or a six-year program in medicine, and after 12 years of schooling. Most of these doctors now practice medicine in the U.S.

There are several reasons for a suggestion to change the entry requirements for obtaining a medical degree. The reasons are economic, societal, and human. On the economic front, this reform would save healthcare costs, because most people who graduate from medical schools end up with an enormous amount of debt. They exhaust their resources in a four-year undergraduate degree program and then proceed to medical school with several loans. This thus increases the total cumulative cost over a period of eight years. Simple economic theory proves that people tend to maximize their return on investment. This increases the expectation for a large salary. Now let us examine how this translates into reality.

Rural areas where 20 percent of the population lives are served only by only 9 percent of the nation's physicians.[10] Inner cities are similarly underserved.[11] All together, of the 738,000 physicians in the United States in 1996, 600,000 (81 percent) were engaged in patient care.[12] Of these, almost 70 percent were specialists.[13] For the year 2000, it is predicted that the number of physicians caring for patients will increase to 203 per 100,000 population, as compared with 115 per 100,000 in 1970.[14] This growth in physician-to-population ratio is attributable to increased number of specialists. This is evidence that there is an oversupply of specialists.

This does raise several questions. The current system of a cumulative eight-year program to become a physician discourages doctors from working in rural areas due to the poor pay scales which limits their ability to meet their financial obligations. Thus we have a system of education that increases the demand for high pay because of the up-front eight-year investment. From a simple perspective of income maximization, most physicians tend to become specialists. Whatever parameters were set forth by medical schools to admit medical students into Universities obviously do not seem to be working.

I recommend that we consider switching to a system like England, where people can obtain a medical degree after high school. The Government can extend the residency training requirements or choose to leave it the same. Both of these dual objectives will lower healthcare costs, keep pay scales in balance, will not encourage more people to become specialists, and may entice more idealistic young people to practice medicine uniformly across several parts of the country, both rural and urban.

REFORMING PATENT LAW

Most people question the high prices for prescription drugs. However, as a nation we may be missing the point. What we should be questioning instead is why and how we got here in the first place. Surprisingly, there is no economic research on the subject of how the current patent law affects the price for prescription pharmaceuticals, and the behavior of the pharmaceutical industry in general.

This is the theory: most products including prescription drugs are provided patent protection for twenty years. However, the effective patent life for pharmaceutical products could range from a few to a maximum of twenty years, usually in the range of 7 through 15 or so years, depending on when the product finally hits the market after the completion of all required studies and the usual approval process. After the drug goes off patent, generic manufacturers produce these drugs at a substantially reduced cost. After patents have expired for important pharmaceutical products, pharmaceutical manufacturers scramble to come out with newer technologies in an effort to produce new drugs in both similar and dissimilar disease classes. New technologies replace old technologies due to the marketing prowess of most of these companies.

In healthcare, sometimes these newer technologies may be beneficial, but at other times they may not necessarily be beneficial. This unintentional encouragement provided by the Government for the replacement of older technologies may have contributed to the high costs of healthcare. The availability of a generic drug does not necessarily mean that they get utilized, because these drugs are not promoted to physicians and have a tendency to be forgotten. Also, the creativity of the drug manufacturers (the effect) and the patent law (the cause) may create the perception in society that the older technologies are less helpful. This is sometimes true and sometimes not true.

One could argue that if the government and the GATT had patent policies on a product line basis (implying a longer life span on patents for pharmaceuticals, especially in crowded therapeutic markets), then the industry would not have come out with new drug entities as rapidly as they would have in the present climate. Competition would have driven the costs of these drugs downwards and the managed care industry with their sophisticated formulary control mechanisms are able to significantly drive the costs down for prescription pharmaceuticals. The cumulative amount of expenses could have been lower due to the absence of "shorter-duration" patent laws on pharmaceuticals and hence may not have forced manufacturers to innovate as rapidly as they would have desired to do so.

If reform was implemented, to allow a patent to have a long life, say, 30 plus years; incentives would be weighted towards developing a new drug only if the company felt there was a true breakthrough in technology. Incentives would instead shift to improving the existing drug. Research would focus on enhancing the value of existing drugs that have already proven to be successful, while decreasing the cost of risk associated with more rapid innovations. It is possible that under such a scenario the cumulative costs for the development of a drug, including the total amount of clinical trials and the associated marketing expense would have been drastically reduced.

On the contrary, we now have a patent law system that geometrically increases costs by providing incentives to "reinvent the wheel" once every seven, eight, twelve years, or fifteen years. Developing a single new drug molecule could take $300-$800 million in research alone, not to mention the costs of marketing these products. Further research and simulation is warranted on how shorter and/or longer duration patent laws increase and/or decrease healthcare costs. If we can not address these issues, it can be expected that in the near future we will be developing more drug entities at an even more rapid pace than today not necessarily to improve healthcare but rather to cope with the issue of declining patents. Therefore, I recommend the system evaluate changing the current patent law system to offer patents on medicines that are much longer term, beyond the typical 20 years. For example, should patents on medicines be similar to copyright laws in crowded disease classes? Medicines are not gadgets, they are a product of long and arduous research requiring more intense human experiments and manual processes than automated gadgets. Therefore, patent protection, long lasting patent life, and customization of patent law by product line may warrant further research.

While we certainly need to civilize free-market economics through an approach that provides balance and harmony to all concerned parties. At the same time, it behooves us to better predict the consequences of our laws and regulations by undertaking a small-scale experiment on providing a longer patent life for medications in crowded and targeted disease classes. For orphan drugs, it is understandable to retain the current patent law structure due to monopolization. However, we have not dared to challenge or experiment on the type of patent law that works and does not work. When the problem is with the root of the tree, we shouldn't be spending too much time in prescribing medicine to the leaves.

In our system, the older and cheaper generics have a minimal place in the society. Whether we like it or not, marketing and innovation will change these dynamics (due to existing patent law). The only way to reduce research and development costs, marketing expenses, and peoples' perceptions, is to think of some radical ways on how patent laws affect healthcare costs. Nobody knows for certain whether the current system of drug patents has increased or decreased drug costs, but we should begin asking the right questions. It is my opinion that they may have increased prescription drug costs because of their shorter effective life spans.

Government and industry must allow innovation to occur in a natural manner and may want to consider allowing patent protection for a longer time duration, atleast in more crowded and targeted disease class as an experiment. Government must and should take an active role in ensuring the safety of medicines, ethical practices, and the safety of its citizens. However, the involvement of the government in a market-based economy may need careful exploration before implementation of major policies. It is hypothesized that patent laws may have contributed to an accelerated pace of drug innovation. As a result, they may have increased the cumulative costs of drug discovery, drug development, and the associated marketing expenses connected with the marketing of new medications. The recent recall of several medications in the areas of diabetes, cardiovascular disease, weight-loss, etc., are clear examples that new innovations in healthcare are not necessarily effective. In the last four years (1997-2000), 10 prescription drugs and a vaccine have been taken off the market after killing and injuring thousands of people.[15] The safety withdrawals of 11 pharmaceuticals in four years appears to be unprecedented. Only eight prescription drugs were pulled for safety reasons in the previous 26 years [16]. Rapid innovations in a compressed time do not necessarily mean newer technologies are always better than the old ones. It is possible that patent laws have put more pressure on companies to innovate and commercialize medicines to maintain shareholder value and stay in business. These high costs associated with offset of "shorter time duration" patent laws may have increased the overall costs of healthcare.

Current shorter time duration patent laws may have also contributed to higher increases in the sales force size of different pharmaceutical companies. When patent laws that provide short product life cycles are replaced with a collaborative partnership between government and industry on post-market safety monitoring it may provide better outcomes for the society as whole. On the contrary, we have created a system that fosters an artificial and an accelerated speed in innovation due to shorter patent life. As a society we should opt for a natural speed in innovation rather than an artificial or a forced speed in drug innovation. Let us learn more clearly the dynamics of existing drugs before we take big leaps in innovating newer drugs.

It would be fair to suggest that reform in patent law may also want to be simultaneously accompanied by questioning a system in which large employers get tax breaks for providing insurance and paying other large organizations such as HMOs and Insurers directly. Transferring tax breaks to individuals would dramatically shift the balance of power to the consumer and will automatically force every company to cater to the needs of smart shoppers. This has been one of the recommendations of the Citizens Against Government Waste that voices the opinions of its 600,000 membership base.[17]

If the computer industry had several manual processes similar to the drug industry, computer costs would have probably increased, and not decreased. We now have better and faster computers with lower costs simply due to automation that is not achievable in healthcare. Industries are unique and product lines within an industry are unique. However, the time duration on patents is similar for most product lines. This is the critical dilemma that needs debate, research, and discussion.

6

Re-engineering Medicare—An Approach to its Solvency

The purpose of this essay is to suggest ideas that will improve the current system of administering Medicare to the 40 million senior citizens in America. The focus of these ideas will be an application of free market principles or privatization concepts to Medicare; streamlining the administration of the current Medicare system; introducing a market based mechanism for financing Medicare and; encouraging market forces to shape the delivery of health care to older Americans.

As the Baby Boom generation approaches retirement age, Medicare, in its current form, is projected to go bankrupt by 2015.[1] In 1970, about 20 million people were covered by this entitlement program. Today that number has nearly doubled. By 2011, more than 77 million people will be eligible for benefits, and by 2040, 81 million people are expected to participate. Spending on behalf of Medicare beneficiaries increased from $21.5 billion in 1977 to $214.6 billion in 1997.[2] However, the full-time, equivalent staff on the agency has remained about the same, at roughly 4,000 people. [3]

The present discussions on modernizing Medicare are either piecemeal or address short-term solutions. At the Congressional level, it has become a game of budget surplus management. At the Medicare administration level, it has become a game of confusion, complication, and consternation. Thus far, no discussion has been centered on getting to the heart of the matter that provides an all-encompassing system of care. Bureaucracy has smothered free market ambition, energy, and creativity to find solutions to the national problem.

There are two key issues with respect to the current state of Medicare: the source of and the application of the Medicare trust fund. The nature of sourcing and the adequate growth of the Medicare trust fund are key issues that merit national debate. Additional debate needs to focus on the appropriate utilization of these funds.

The fundamental question that needs to be addressed is: How can we enable Medicare operate like any other business or a public company? The Medicare Trust Fund must be utilized to bring about growth, similar to the returns achieved by the top quartile of a balanced mutual fund. Also, the Health Care Financing Administration (HCFA) now called as the Center for Medicaid & Medicare Services (CMS) must adopt the role of a corporate employer, wherein the corporate employer purchases healthcare on behalf of its employees and does not get involved in establishing elaborate price setting mechanisms for managed care. At the present time, Medicare is complicated because the government and HCFA have assumed multiple roles. These roles include the role of a corporate employer, HMO, physician, hospital, Long Term Care Provider, etc. Interwoven with these roles are an experimentation of the concepts utilized in Europe and Canada. This has thus created a system of bureaucracy that has rippled through the entire managed care industry to create several layers of administration. The Congressional leaders talk about reducing administrative costs on one hand, but at the same time all of their actions are indicative of increasing costs.

BACKGROUND

The CMS administers Medicare, the nation's largest health insurance program, covering over 40 million Americans at an annual cost of about $200 billion.[4] Medicare provides health insurance to all people who are at least 65 years old. Medicare is composed of two parts: Hospital Insurance (Part A) and Medical Insurance (Part B).

- **Medicare Part A:** provides coverage of inpatient hospital services, skilled nursing facilities, home health services, and hospice care.

- **Medicare Part B:** helps pay for the cost of physician services, outpatient hospital services, medical equipment and supplies, and other health services and supplies.

In broad terms, Medicare offers a fee-for-service arrangement (the original Medicare plan that is available to everyone) and the Medicare+Choice plan, which is a Medicare Managed Care Plan available in many parts of the country. In 1999, Preferred Provider Organizations, Provider Sponsored Organizations, and other insurance options like Private-Fee-For-Service Plans and Medicare Medical Savings Accounts also became available. No matter what option a Medicare recipient chooses, they are still in the Medicare program and will receive at least all of the basic Medicare covered services.

FINANCING ISSUES

Let us first review the current manner in which Medicare operates from a financial perspective. These may be broadly viewed from two different angles.

a. How does the government support Medicare? (Where does the money come from?)

b. How does it support/finance the delivery of care (Medicare) through CMS? (How is the money utilized to provide healthcare?)

Let us briefly evaluate parts (a) and (b) and then provide some ideas on how they may potentially be improved.

a. The Federal government finances the current system of Medicare through a collection of Medicare taxes. The National Bipartisan Commission a group convened by the Federal Government to examine Medicare has had several debates on modernizing Medicare. The media has expressed numerous concerns on the future solvency of Medicare. These activities have helped start a national conversation, even among the general public. The proposal promoted by the National Bipartisan Commission did not provide necessary revenues to protect Medicare's future. In fact, it passed up a historic chance to dedicate part of our budget surplus directly to the program. The former President, Bill Clinton, wanted to reserve 15 percent of our surplus just for Medicare, which would shore up the trust fund until 2027.

The Commission's proposal was also a factor in the rise of the Medicare eligibility age, but it failed to protect those who would be left without coverage. In that sense, there is concern that it would make the lack of insurance problem for older Americans worse, not better.

The proposal also did not provide a workable solution for providing prescription drug benefits for all Medicare beneficiaries. Estimates are that half of Medicare beneficiaries spend over $500 on drugs in just one year, some as much as a thousand. And over one-third do not have private coverage to help pay for the drugs that they need to stay healthy.

b. The CMS has an elaborate system for financing Medicare. In addition to financing Medicare recipients in a fee-for-service environment, the agency also has the responsibility of financing the delivery of care in the managed care environment. About six million of the 40 million Medicare recipients are now enrolled in managed care.[5] CMS finances the delivery of this care in a variety of ways. It utilizes a competitive bidding process, in which suppliers submit bids and Medicare selects only the lowest cost bids that provide the best price and quality. This promotes a "center of excellence" concept, in which hospitals and doctor groups that meet high quality standards are paid a single bundled payment for all services related to specific and complex procedures. With respect to managed care, the newly implemented Balanced Budget Act (BBA) provisions will reallocate HMO reimbursements in rural and urban areas. Before BBA, HMO reimbursement rates were based entirely on fee-for-service costs in their local area. This means that HMOs in lower-cost rural areas receive lower payments than those in higher-cost urban areas. Under the BBA, plan rates will be based on a combination—or "blend"—of local and national rates. This budget-neutral "blend" will help encourage the development of managed care plans by increasing reimbursement rates in lower cost, rural areas where many Medicare enrollees have limited managed care choices. With respect to home health or long term care, CMS administers the Prospective Payment System (PPS). Suffice it to say that all of these governmental price fixing mechanisms have added more complexity to the managed care industry.

There are inherent deficiencies in both (a) and (b) as noted above. First, regarding (a), I recommend that the taxes collected under Medicare be put to good use to ensure an adequate and reasonable return on the money. For example, the money should be invested in a manner that would produce a return equivalent to a well-established balanced mutual fund. Investing 50 percent in stocks and 50 percent in bonds may be a good compromise and may help Medicare assure solvency, this view was expressed by some economists and the former President Bill Clinton.

With respect to (b) the government must decide to move away from a "centralized" approach of financing care under Medicare to a more "decentralized" approach. The present method of financing care under Medicare by CMS is centralized and creates parallel systems of administration both by CMS and the managed care industry. The managed care industry includes HMOs and the senior care industry, example, the long term care institutions and home health. Most HMOs have designed parallel systems in addition to their existing systems simply to increase enrollment of the Medicare recipients or satisfy the needs of CMS. Randall Brown and Marsha Gold at the Mathematica Policy Research in Princeton, New Jersey, say that state regulations have altered the direction of managed care growth.[6] They further cite that the States' reporting requirements have added to costs, and restrictions on marketing and pricing have inhibited a plans' ability to promote their products and secure competitive rates for services.[7] They conclude that in order to prudently shape Medicare managed care, policy makers need to focus less on national statistics and more on local market variations.[8] Many reformers believe that the use of market forces is a more effective means of controlling health-spending growth than the current regulatory methods. These reformers have touted the Federal Employees Health Benefit Program (FEHBP) as a model for reforming Medicare. The most advantageous feature of this program is that premiums are established in the market.

For all of these reasons, both the Government and HMOs would benefit tremendously if the Government completely scrapped or re-engineered its present method of payment and reimbursement rates through several complex formulas. Government should treat HMOs as true "Centers of Excellence," and must allow HMOs to determine premium rates for enrolling Medicare recipients. HMOs are more in touch with the day-to-day business and the local market variations. This concept is no different than HMOs providing premium rates for employer groups. Therefore, based on this recommendation, the role of CMS would change from that of a centralized agency determining pre-established rates to one where CMS acts as any other employer group in the country, accepting and deciding between competitive rates offered by several managed care institutions. CMS, like an employer, would now be able to obtain the best competitive rate from competing HMOs. It is also recommended that CMS, or a revamped

CMS, function as a corporate business to obtain the best possible rate of return on the money that it collects from working Americans as Medicare taxes.

ADMINISTRATIVE RATIONALE FOR MODERNIZING MEDICARE

The changes suggested above have the potential to radically change Medicare by shifting power from the Government to the market. American business history has always proven that when decisions are de-centralized to the market place, it encourages innovation and efficiency. This is not to say that HMOs are perfect, however, they are trying to become more efficient.

Information technology will ultimately help make things efficient. "We spend $1.2 trillion on health care,—$450 billion on administrative costs," says former Senator Bill Bradley. "By simply moving things from paper to the Internet, you will be able to achieve significant savings."[9] A recent study by the consulting firm Deloitte & Touche found that the healthcare industry spends just $2,800 per year per employee on information technology.[10] By contrast, retailers spend $5,700, the oil-and-gas industry $8,800 and banks $10,400.[11] This shows that healthcare is terribly far behind other industries in adopting information technology. CMS and the Government must not compound these problems by creating parallel systems of financing healthcare. Such parallel systems of financing healthcare will only increase costs in the long term and could create more confusion in the industry in the form of consolidations, increases in premium rates in the non-Medicare sector, etc. Just imagine translating a 130,000-page Medicare document on a computer.

According to an October 2000 study by a medical researcher at Northwest Healthcare Networks, it costs HMOs an average of $10 per patient to make an appointment on the internet versus $70 over the phone.[12] This is just one example of how information technology could reduce administrative costs. In the long run, administrative costs can only be streamlined in healthcare if the existence of multiple financing systems, pricing options, and choices are also streamlined. Both the Government and the managed care industry must make a concerted effort in this direction. This is true for almost all systems of healthcare including hospital systems, physician visits, or prescription drugs. Medical, scientific, pharmaceutical, technological and actuarial innovations have added to the bureaucracy in healthcare. In the long run, however, all of these innovations are necessary. Healthcare is still in the formative stage where people are groping for the right answers or for the right business model. Free markets have always proven that answers eventually do arise and profits are equitably distributed. For example, prior to the birth of Pharmacy Benefit Management (PBM) companies, retail pharmacies were dispensing prescriptions with high mark-ups somewhere in the range of 5-35 percent on average above the Average Wholesale Price (AWP) of the prescription. However, when entrepreneurs started experimenting with PBM companies, the retail pharmacies had to forego these mark-ups and the profits ultimately were funneled back to the different sectors, including employer groups or plan sponsors of pharmacy care.

While healthcare has standardized some innovations, it has also tended to accommodate many other innovations with minimal standardization. For example, there is little standardization among insurers' record-keeping systems. As a result, doctors who deal with multiple health plans must submit information in many different formats before they can be confident that bills will be paid. In this case the Federal Government has directed insurers to standardize their approaches. It is exactly this kind of role that the Federal Government needs to play—even in the case of Medicare—to channel, streamline, and standardize innovations in healthcare before they go out of control and further increase healthcare costs.

Chief Executive David M. Lawrence of Kaiser Permanente, the country's largest HMO, launched a massive $2 billion project to move all of its operations to the Internet. He plans to create digital medical records for each of Kaiser's 9 million members and to electronically link its 361 hospitals and clinics with Kaiser's 10,000 doctors, nurses, and dentists. He also plans to set up customized websites so that major clients can look up their particular rates or coverage. In the Northwest region of Kaiser, where the Internet system has been in place for two years, Kaiser's costs increased at a 2.1 percent pace in 1999, down from a six percent average annual rate in the mid-1990's.[13] And only three of Kaiser's six regional divisions are using the Internet system to date. Kaiser is one of the most technologically savvy HMOs. In general, most of the healthcare industry lags behind in information technology. "I don't think the healthcare industry overall has figured out the benefits of the Internet," says David Wachpress, director of undergraduate e-commerce programs at the New Jersey Institute of Technology.[14]

Now imagine the Kaiser scenario, and add to it a separate wrinkle on administering Medicare rates at different institutions and figure out the extra investment in hardware, software and manpower. This is how we complicate healthcare. Introducing principles that have been successful elsewhere into a free market system, such as ours, can hamper the very components of the American free enterprise system that have created value time and again through experimentation.

The $450 billion healthcare administrative costs that Bradley speaks of are simply due to the plethora of choices and complexities that we have introduced into the healthcare system. Take, for example, the current debate on prescription drugs. Should Medicare decide to institute a centralized system on obtaining the lowest possible price for a drug, then Medicare will have created a new administrative system that ripples through the managed care industry—HMOs would have to create new systems with pharmaceutical manufacturers to administer pharmaceutical rebates separately for Medicare recipients, and HMOs would have to create an additional software system to funnel these savings back to Medicare. The pharmaceutical manufacturers also would need to create additional systems to administer these contracts, thus complicating existing systems even further. However, if the Government transferred the complete onus of the Medicare administration to managed care plans, similar to what employers do, savings would be significant. All CMS or the Government would have to do is to obtain competitive rates from the managed care industry. When both the Government and managed care industry drive towards standardization in health care, then and only then savings in health care will be achieved. The current system of Medicare is unfortunately heading more towards non-standardization in the industry and will create additional costs in almost every sector, including pharmaceuticals.

Information technology in and of itself is not a cure for all ills. Information technology can be utilized to increase or decrease administrative costs. If information technology is utilized to provide fanciful packaging to healthcare, it has the potential to increase costs. The challenge for the healthcare industry is to use technology to decrease administrative costs, a plethora of product options, healthcare delivery schemes, and pricing mechanisms that sometimes expand consumer choice only to cause confusion, yet they all parade under the shibboleth of "choice." When these choices are not streamlined, they burden the healthcare system and become accepted norms. Finding the right balance is the key to achieving optimum cost efficiencies both in administration and operating costs of the healthcare industry in general.

CONTRIBUTING A PERCENTAGE OF LIFE INSURANCE POLICY TO MEDICARE

If the Government is serious about containing costs for Medicare, we have to think in ingenious ways like Thomas Edison. Edison's original business model for electricity required customers to pay a flat fee for connection to the network. He soon realized that the dramatic difference in wealth between his first customer, the mighty J.P. Morgan Bank, and his subsequent, small-business customers necessitated a more flexible model, so he invented a device to measure electricity use and charged accordingly.

Today, we have all Medicare recipients under a similar scheme, regardless of wealth status, pay the same premium and avail of the same services. Therefore, it makes sense that we think like Edison and let the free markets come up with solutions on designing the healthcare meters. The Government would be wise to hand over the reins of the healthcare delivery system completely to the managed care industry. The Federal Government should be an active partner in the process, without interference, similar to the Employer/HMO interface. Markets are sometimes self-correcting and in the long run wealth may get distributed equitably. Should this not happen, the Government has the right to correct this process through enacting laws or rules. One example of an idea for a healthcare meter would be for a Medicare recipient to "sign-off," a portion of his or her life insurance death benefits to Medicare, based on certain defined parameters.

Most beneficiaries who require medical care receive far more from the program than they contributed in payroll taxes. Overall, 89 percent of Medicare's revenue now comes primarily from people who are less than 65 years old, through payroll taxes, income taxes, and interest on the trust fund, and 11 percent comes from the monthly premiums contributed by the elderly beneficiaries. From a cash flow perspective, more money leaves the system than is taken in, and the problem will only be exacerbated—unless we devise a system whereby a life insurance death benefit of a specified amount or percentage, depending on the wealth status of an individual, goes to the Government. If the Government has taken care of a Medicare recipient in a nursing home for an extended period of time, it is reasonable that the Government will be left with a bequest, especially if the individual was wealthy with a decent life insurance policy. In the future, the system cannot survive if only the young have to support the old. A variety of ideas have to be blended in a seamless fashion, these ideas can only spring from diverse places, and the role of the Government must be to take leadership to weave these ideas together and leave innovation to the industry. When the Government acts as an innovator, it ends up becoming a regulator and strangles innovation.

OPINION RESEARCH

Medicare senior citizens are the ultimate customers of any system they belong to. Their satisfaction and opinions on the future of Medicare must also be taken into account. Given the complex nature of Medicare, the Medicare debate with seniors included must be in the context of vision, information, and right knowledge. The focus of the debate has to be on the "system" as opposed to "pieces of the system." The CareData and Sachs/Scarborough Healthplus surveys show that greater than 70 percent of the Medicare enrollees are satisfied with their enrollment in HMOs.[15] The Sachs survey included about 3.5 million people. These surveys are not to sanction HMOs, or to conclude that they have been successful, for it is only one approach. There are examples where the Program of All-Inclusive Care for the Elderly (PACE) have been quite successful to reduce both Medicare and Medicaid expenditures. It has been touted as a model that needs to be emulated. [16]

Finally, the pattern of maturation of the behemoth that is the American healthcare industry has resulted in a concoction of the free enterprise and socialist systems. We have allowed the high cost of medical malpractice insurance, trial lawyers, and unlimited damages flourish in some components of the healthcare system and have tightly regulated some other components. Legal lawsuits in every area have become the first resort instead of being the last. A red flag should be raised if the debate seeks out for the best of both worlds. We either resort to a system like in Britain and Canada or pursue the American way. We must be open to ideas, but let ideas be compatible and transmutable so that the system works like a frictionless machine.

CONCLUSION

It is important that the nation focus the Medicare debate on the important structural changes needed for the entire system, including Medicare and its interface with the entire healthcare industry. These are more specific to the growth of the trust fund, the correct application of these funds without increasing administrative costs in the entire health-care system, and ensuring that people pay according to their needs and individual wealth status. I am certain managed care will take up the challenge on designing the appropriate systems. Innovation and creativity are born among people and diversity, however, they are not born in pedantic political debates or bipartisan commissions. One never knows what the outcome will look like, but at least we know it will be more positive because it would be an application of free market principles with the Government taking the lead on the will to change, and all parties committing themselves in a sincere attempt to address the needs of the elderly. The Medicare debate will succeed if the focus is on the entire system rather than on specific components of the system. We need to lock in the debate on the philosophy and direction rather than on political and media demagogue.

PART IV

7

Stress, Organizational Design, Social innovations and Long Term Effects on Health and Costs

The relationship between stress and the workplace has received considerable attention in the media. The true price tag of stress alone to healthcare costs is unknown. In 1993, The United Nations International Labor Organization estimated that U.S. industry lost about $200 billion due to job related stress.[1]

STRESS, HEALTH, AND PRODUCTIVITY

The growing demands for productivity in the workplace, the need for assimilation and dissemination of growing information, the ability for both men and women to balance obligation between work and family, and the anxiety to maintain a level of prosperity combined with a tension of insecurity between personal lives and work lives, all exacerbate stress differently for different individuals. This difference is based on our ability to cope with stress based on how we allow the external and the internal physiological environments to challenge us. For some individuals, stress is a lesson-learned, they learn as much from their misery as they learn from happiness. For other individuals, extreme forms of stress can drive them to substance abuse. Again, stress is a function of our capacity to better cope with external events—good or bad.

From the point of view of an individual, the only way to control stress is to look at the causes of stress itself with a positive attitude. This is because chronic stress can be disruptive to ones health, as the regulation of several essential hormones when disturbed over long periods of time lead to diseases such as stroke, hypertension, and heart disease. The sayings "the world is a hard place to live in" and that "life is not fair" are true. These things will always be given. Happiness and misery have never disappeared from the world, they only keep evolving and mesmerizing us in their cyclical twists and turns. In United States and Europe, researchers have found little if any correlation between income and happiness. Being happy or less stressed is only a state of mind. There are now a plethora of books on the subject of stress and happiness. The purpose of this chapter is not to discuss stress or offer a long essay on happiness; the important point, however, is that we should not blame others for our stress. This further accentuates the very basis of stress itself. We must become creative in dealing with our stress. Depending on our own nature, we can either fight stress through internal will power or, as circumstances warrant, we can change our external environment through the right means. For example, a person living in a dictatorial regime cannot go out and assassinate their leader. On the other hand, in the same regime, a creative person would have found a different way to cope with his stress, either adjusting to his environment or taking a leadership approach to foster democracy.

Fate plays a negligible role in controlling stress or being happy. The mechanism of adaptation explains why people can be happy after physically disabling tragedies. Therefore, our ability to cope with stress and being happy is truly a state of mind. For our own health and our own pocketbook, we need to learn on how to deal with stress and just be happy.

Obviously, the question that arises is why shouldn't individuals resign themselves to their situation and be happy? Unfortunately, this is not the very nature of human beings. Individual growth depends upon the fulfillment of ones desires. Fulfillment of desires brings happiness, further raising our aspirations for future desires. Frustration usually sets in when our desires are not fulfilled. This frustration causes stress. Most organizations and businesses realize this kind of stress and constantly try to provide opportunities for people to grow and relieve their frustrations. Most organizations are familiar with job-related stress. Transitioning from an individual's ability to cope with stress, let us examine what organizations can and can not do to alleviate the stress of its employees.

Some organizations try to lower stress through better organizational design, and others through programs. Most, however, foster a culture where people can grow and fulfill their desires. Provided below are some concepts that organizations may have overlooked.

When power remains at the top, it causes more stress at the bottom—it limits the ability of employees to grow. Extreme examples are dictatorial regimes that have existed in several countries and continue to exist even in the new millennium. This stress at the bottom has resulted in revolts and revolutions. On the other extreme, is our own culture in the U.S. the vision of Thomas Jefferson, who penned the profound expression our culture is founded on, "Life, Liberty, and the Pursuit of Happiness," the wisdom of the founding fathers allows individuals to grow and express their creativity. Had the founding fathers kept all the power for themselves, the country and its citizens would not have achieved or realized the present state of its growth. Therefore, people in organizations too will become more powerful by relinquishing their power—power must be decentralized to the lowest possible unit. It will be an organizational manifestation of life, liberty, and the pursuit of happiness. This decentralization of power may reduce stress at every level of any corporation. Organizations must redesign themselves to become consistent with this concept. The desires of a company to make a difference in people's lives depends on the continuous challenges and opportunities they provide to make all levels of people empowered.

According to Dr. Joyce Brothers, one of the world's most well-known psychologists, "Happy people aren't necessarily the busiest people, but they're usually busy with things they feel enthusiastic about."[2] She further concludes that when people are intensely involved in an activity they like, total engagement produces a sense of contentment that makes the person doing the task, and the task at hand, become one. In a nutshell, organizational design is all about generating the optimal amount of enthusiasm for individuals or groups of individuals. This design must be focused around the general areas of interest that serve both business objectives and produce an experience for the employees where there is a state of absolute absorption. Organizations of the future will survive by not seeking to get a job done, but rather by seeking to ensure that an individual employee is contented.

When we show respect to all individuals, regardless of their level in a corporation, they feel empowered. When we as individuals learn to give away our power, we become more powerful. Decentralization of power to the next lower unit does not make us "less" but makes us "more" powerful. This thus contributes to less stress in the organization because we become aware of satisfying the emotional needs of everyone in the organization. Happiness does not come solely from desires being fulfilled; it comes from emotional needs being met. Getting what we want is gratifying. Leadership does not gratify, true leadership provides satisfaction to employees. It makes people know that their work is appreciated and their work has a place in the world. It is important that we do not lose sight of the true meaning of work and vision. Work and vision are truly correlated with a mission. This enhances the dignity of the worker and the corporation. This is echoed in the oft-quoted sentence from the British thinker, the late Bernard Shaw: " This is the true joy in life—to be used for a purpose which you consider mighty; to be a force in nature, and not a clod of ailments and grievances, ever complaining that the world does not devote itself to making you happy."[3]

When organizations learn to function with a mission, respect for customers increases. Therefore, an organization grows and contributes to the further growth of its employees. When organizations tend to follow such a path, they can expect their healthcare costs to be impacted favorably due to lowered levels of stress.

I would also like to state that the closer organizations are connected to their vision (mission), the more its people will take pride in their work. This pride decreases stress due to increased fulfillment of employees emotional needs or desires. The innate nature of most human beings working for corporations is to benefit society. Therefore, it is natural that the closer a company is to its vision, the closer it will fulfill the desires of its employees, as well as society.

STRESS IN CHILDREN AND ITS LONG TERM EFFECTS ON HEALTH

One couldn't start this section without thinking of the famous maxim of Benjamin Franklin, "Early to bed, early to rise, makes a man (person) healthy, wealthy and wise." Let us see how this proverb plays out among our youth and how it impacts their thinking and health as they grow older.

In the last one hundred years, we have seen several important achievements: two world wars, the invention of radio, the television, automobiles, motorcycles, airplanes, spaceships, and satellites, the industrial revolution, sending a man to the moon, nuclear power, unfolding of the many secrets of the universe, several high-tech innovations in every area of physical and medical science, the computer revolution, the internet revolution, the mapping of the human genome, several financial innovations, medical innovations, economic innovations, and many more. Most people feel we compressed time unlike our predecessors, or that we have lived several centuries in one short century.

Our institutions, our culture, and our enterprise have made these phenomena happen. As we move forward, we want our children to progress in a similar manner—from a "fast forward," motion of the twentieth century to a "super fast forward," motion of the twenty-first century. Our beliefs and attitudes shaped the twentieth century. We therefore would want the twenty-first century to proceed at a much faster pace. Universal time may be eternal, but our time is certainly not eternal. Our youth understand very well the culture we live and work in.

It is my belief that most high school and college-bound students sleep normally beyond 11 p.m. and sometimes even after 12 p.m. In the present day and age, the wisdom of Benjamin Franklin, "Early to bed and early to rise makes a body healthy, wealthy, and wise," is considered old-fashioned wisdom. The current belief is that if we want to compete in the new age, we need to forget about old proverbs. Unfortunately, this thinking has been exported to the outside world as well. These cultures now challenge us by competing with us on the ground rules that we established. All of this has now led to a competitive vicious cycle, an age where the competition of minds and brainpower reigns supreme. Nowadays, measly stock returns of 10 percent are considered poor returns: we are not satisfied until we see greater than 10– 20 percent average stock market returns every year, and this is the culture that we may be slowly trying to disseminate the world over. Therefore, from now on, global technological progress will continue at an even more rapid pace. This progress will come at the cost of our health and of the health of our children. We all parade under the shibboleth of fast progress: achieving everything in a compressed time and seeking to tap ever more from nature than giving back it back. We wonder about the root causes of our illnesses, when the solutions are right in front of us. Thus we ended the twentieth century with further newfound chronic illnesses such as Attention Deficit and Hyperactivity

Disorders (ADHD), Chronic Fatigue Syndrome, etc. These illnesses are growing at an alarming rate and are more pronounced among children and adolescents especially in the technologically developed countries.[4] Several adults are also experiencing these illnesses. For ADHD we have drug therapies such as Ritalin, but these therapies have serious side effects. For chronic fatigue, industry will find a cure that may require less sleep for an individual. Eventually, we may even trace these illnesses to defective genes. We may even begin to define health and regulate it as a commodity. We will likely find cures for such illnesses through drugs, since this is an easy way out. If our tendencies to seek solutions at the top-end continue, our healthcare costs will also increase. We certainly need to define our limits, if we truly want to contain our healthcare costs. Trying to address our problems by utilizing a bottoms-up approach will reveal to us that these problems may not be in our genes but rather the way in which we ruin our genes. Unless we address the problems that beset humanity, the nature of our educational system, the complex interactive processes of society, etc., we may only increase and not decrease our healthcare costs. Seeking a top-down approach to solutions is a mind-engaging, intellectually delightful game of fixes and manipulations that usually results in more sophisticated bureaucracy. Let us not water the leaves when it is the root that needs the watering.

Only when technological progress is balanced with social innovation, will we move at the right speed and export the right leadership. We need to ask ourselves whether our education system focuses on the training of the mind at the expense of our inner growth. The former for the most part has a tendency to accelerate complex solutions to complex problems fraught with more dangers. Whereas a focus on the latter may provide simple solutions to complex problems that have less dangers associated with them. This approach in the long term lowers costs in every field, not only healthcare. We need only study the lives of great people to test the validity of these statements. It is the Christ, the Buddha, or the Krishna who are remembered for a millenium—the triumph of wisdom and spirit over pure intellect has survived the test of several thousand centuries. Once we realize this, we will realize that bodies don't suffer, it is people who suffer. People are not just genetic lego bricks of tissues wrapped up in skin. We are more than our genes, and more than our body. Once we realize this, we will embrace an open-mindedness that seeks to address our healthcare issues in an all embracing manner of body, mind, and spirit.

Bill Joy, Chief Scientist of Sun Microsystems, once voiced concern about twenty-first century technologies. Joy warns that so-called nanotechnology, the nascent science of making molecule-size machines, could produce plagues of tiny self replicating robots capable of obliterating life as we know it-or worse, allow high powered computers to think and, therefore, destroy. "My optimism leads to my concern. There could be easily be tens of thousands of dot-geno, dot-nano, dot-robo companies creating trillions of dollars of wealth. The downside: We're on the cusp of further perfection of ...an evil whose possibility spreads well beyond that which weapons of mass destruction bequeathed to the nation states...(it is) just too much for a species at our level of sophistication."[5] This captures in a nutshell the extremes of good news, bad news story—complex solutions to complex problems, a testament and challenge on the accomplishment of our intellect and not of our spirit.

Does this mean we should turn the clock backwards? Certainly not, but we do need to temper our rapid progress with social innovations. This will reduce stress in society and will contain long-term increases in the costs of healthcare. Our universities and schools should take up the challenge of training the mind, body and spirit. Our very foundation of education is headed towards a lopsided growth of our personalities. We deem it to be progress. The side effects of this progress will be geometrically proportional to the perceived advances it may create. The progress we foresee is a creation of a fantasy-land, but if that is what we want, we should expect more increases in our healthcare costs as well. Of late, in the United States, there has been a ten-fold increase in depression, and it is presenting itself at an alarming rate in the early teen years.[6] We are clueless on what accounts for this epidemic in depression when all indexes of objective well-being should point to happiness. Medication and therapy have limits —they may indeed reflect another high cost solution to a problem whose solutions may not be connected to medicine alone. All of these examples will increase healthcare costs, and the cost increases will go beyond healthcare. If we do not address these problems in the right manner, they become, to an extent, a commercial opportunity.

These lopsided approaches on progress are already being plagiarized at an ever more rapid pace in most developing countries, where they are considered fashionable. We are all in a global game that seeks solutions that are outside of ourselves, when, in reality, the solutions are right within us. Our problems will not be solved by high cost technological innovations, we will be forced to turn to low cost social innovations that address and touch our hearts and minds. If we keep this in mind the very foundations of our education will change and will address those good old proverbs of Benjamin Franklin that have more wisdom than all innovations put together...they might just save our health and our lives.

This section is not contradictory to the previous section on organizational design and the fulfillment of desires of individuals. Right now most of our desires are lopsided—rapidly accelerating towards the fulfillment of achieving quick growth to satisfy wealth rather than job satisfaction. People will argue there is nothing wrong with this approach. However, we will know when it is wrong, because organizations will realize that unsafe innovations will fail more quickly because individuals are not tied to a societal vision, they are more tied to a commercial interest. Therefore, it is only right that educational institutions train the total personality of an individual, i.e., their mind, their body, and their spirit. It is only through such methods that organizations will see their true mission and purpose fulfilled, because the costs associated with the risk of innovation itself will be reduced, plus innovations will be a product of wisdom and not just intellect alone. One could even say that they could be low-cost innovations. Chapter 8, provides a practical framework on how such an approach can lower our healthcare costs.

8

Balancing Technological Progress with Social Innovations to Contain Healthcare Costs

Social innovations are those innovations that can be considered life enhancing, life supporting, or even life enriching—they are not necessarily innovations that satisfy our material needs. These innovations certainly improve our total health and provide meaning for our lives. Whether these innovations take place in our personal lives, family lives, in our corporation, our community, our township or city infrastructure, the global landscape or whatever process we interact with, they should all be considered to be within the realm of a social innovation.

Social innovations within the realm of our individual lives relate to our lifestyle, positive and life nurturing belief systems, uplifting thoughts, philosophic or spiritual endeavors, prayer, church, family, etc. Social innovations within corporations may relate to a continuous evaluation of organizational systems, adaptation to a societal mission, improvements to manufacturing processes that replenish nature, etc. Social innovations in education could relate to innovations in character building, understanding the true potential of a human, providing equal emphasis on the development of the physical, mental, and the spiritual aspirations of human beings, etc. The scope of this book is not to provide a dissertation on social innovations, other than to make a point on how they may impact our healthcare costs. Several eminent personalities and thinkers have touched on these areas. However, many of these principles need to be integrated into practice to demonstrate their favorable impact on health. There are innumerable phenomena that we observe in everyday life that are in dire need of social innovation to contain our healthcare costs. I have borrowed an example that is discussed below.

Paul Ehrlich, a Bing Professor of Population Studies and Professor of Biological Sciences at Stanford University, comments in his book *Human Natures*, "It is becoming increasingly clear that cities in countries as diverse as the United States, Mexico, England, China, Australia, and Japan have been or are being designed for the convenience of automobiles rather than people. The results are horrifyingly obvious and similar, but it is virtually impossible to generate a dialog about virtually rehumanizing these societies. Being able to get to work by foot, bicycle, or mass transit not only would greatly benefit our life-supporting systems but also would increase the quality and length of individual lives—not just by reducing pollution and accidental deaths and, in some cases, by increasing exercise but also by reducing the stresses of driving."[1] He further concludes that politicians across the world are still building more highways to relieve traffic congestion, which, as experience around the world has shown, exacerbates rather than solves problems.

This aptly captures my visits to India. The roads in India were never built for automobiles. But now, in several cities across India, politicians build highways to relieve traffic congestion for a dominant middle class that is now equal to the size of the U.S. population. All of these people can afford to buy cars, and, therefore, clog a land system that is about three times the size of Texas. This has caused more pollution, increased the number of asthmatic sufferers, trapped more carbon dioxide, and increased the heat in the region as a whole, thus devastating the overall quality of air, ecosystem, and health.

The hues and dimensions of the application of social innovations are as variegated as the technological innovations that mankind has produced. Social innovations are inconvenient, they are not glamorous, they have no appeal in a world culture that believes in "top-down" solutions and easy fixes. Our education system has never prepared us to address these problems. Our education system has prepared us to live, interact, and succeed in a growth culture where money talks and everything else walks. It would be appropriate to provide some examples on why our system of education is so much focused towards growth at the expense of society. In school biology, we are taught to look at animals as a subject for experimentation. Storytelling is converted to a dry study of anatomical structures. On the contrary, if we looked at these animals as living, conscious beings endowed with mystical powers, maybe we would have protected nature in a better manner. Giant silk moths are not bugs that should be killed, they have the power of being extremely sensitive to low concentrations of chemicals. Dogs have chemoreceptive capabilities to detect the presence of hormones mimicking synthetic chemicals. When people studied the mystical power behind the eyes of a lobster, they created one of the most powerful telescopes in the world. Is there a difference between the health status of animals that subsist on meat versus those that subsist on plant nutrients? What can we learn about organization and management from a colony of ants? Do ants have a better kingdom than us where there seems to be a minimal disparity between their haves and have-nots? How do animals adapt themselves so quickly to nature? Why do animals stretch after their sleep, whereas humans don't seem to follow a similar practice. We just jump out of our beds and get busy. We clearly do not know if this is a healthy practice. Why do some virus and bacteria develop resistance so quickly? Similarly, in physics, what is the nature and relationship between heavenly bodies? Are the macrocosm and the microcosm structured the same?

When the system of education is turned topsy-turvy, and when we study with a purpose and a goal for co-existence with nature, rather than command, dominate, and control, we will have better social innovations. Success and progress are a measure, application, and employment of both of both scientific and humanistic ideas. On a worldwide basis the emphasis has been on command and control. Nature, including the animal kingdom has fostered diversity. Progress is not a one size fits all strategy, every country should not try to mimic another. Countries should learn to complement their core competencies while embracing diversity in thought, word, and deed. The training of humanistic impulses or even developing systems that train the human conscience may be appropriate in the long term. Placing equal emphasis on the physical, mental, and the spiritual aspirations are more appropriate. Such social innovations may be lacking at the present time or are not being adequately tapped.

Most developing countries mimic more opulent lifestyles because these countries are trapped in a culture of over-consumption . All of these desires are now being triggered by the affordability of television and easy access to several different channels across the world. People now want to emulate the lifestyles of their Western counterparts, movie stars, and local media celebrities'.[2] In an overcrowded world, especially in overcrowded countries like India and China, all these factors tax natural capital. Natural capital includes all the familiar resources used by humankind: water, minerals, oil, trees, fish, soil, air, et cetera. But it also encompasses living systems, which include grasslands, savannas, wetlands, estuaries, oceans, coral reefs, riparian corridors, tundras, and rainforests. These countries have already resorted to rationing fresh water, electricity, and other basic necessities. This has further caused several daily stresses in the lives of individuals in these countries. Historically, in most eastern societies, spiritual, public, and private matters integrated and addressed the *whole* of human needs. Unfortunately, they have now disintegrated to more narrow transactions between labor and capital. Paul Hawken, Amory Lovins, & Hunter Lovins, in their book, *Natural Capitalism: Creating the Next Industrial Revolution*, state that for all the world to live as American or

Canadian, we would need two more earths to satisfy everyone, three more still if population should double, and twelve earths altogether if worldwide standards of living should double over the next forty years.[3] They calculate this based on a number of phenomena such as the loss of fresh water ecosystems at the rate of 6 percent per year, marine ecosystems at 4 percent a year, the loss of a fourth of worlds topsoil in the past half century, etc.[4] The intent here is not to predict doom but rather to point out that using resources at a greater rate than they can be replenished may lead to trouble. Human endeavor will always try to find the right solutions by converting problems into opportunities. However, we cannot wait for the problem to worsen.

John Holdren, Anne Ehrlich, and Paul Ehrlich describe the impact of human population on Earth's life support systems by the equation:
I = PAT
Impact, I, is equal to population size, P, multiplied by affluence, A (measured as per capita consumption), in turn multiplied by the technologies, T (including social, political and economic arrangements), that service the consumption. [5]

It is my hypothesis that the higher the "I", or the higher the depletion of natural capital, the higher our increases in healthcare costs, irrespective of country. Social scientists should pursue further research to prove this hypothesis. If found true, employers would now participate more actively in policy and society. This awareness itself could be considered a social innovation. We are all aware that overcrowding in populous countries like India and China brings forth a variety of tropical diseases. It is also possible that habits of overconsumption may have led to marked changes in lifestyles in the Western countries, such as the increase in the rates of cancer and several other chronic diseases. It is likely that future generations could blame the present generation for their destructive lifestyles that may have led to bad genes rather than solely placing the blame on the genes. The blame could be directed at *us* rather than the gene. What if this generation developed proof that genes were simply an expression of our thought and lifestyles, and probably evolved imperfections through destruction of the environment and ecosystems. We are clearly not certain whether this generation would simply accept a quick-fix solution to all of these problems.

Urgently needed is a worldwide social dialog designed to address a new set of rules: the meaning of "economic progress" as a panacea for all our ills will not solve our problems.

The practical way is for all individuals to change, leading to societal change and changing organizations and the entire fabric of society. We need to become trainers and developers of human character and natural capital. When fast competition masquerades as progress there will be side effects and these side effects will increase healthcare costs. Unbeknownst to us, several phenomena, including the depletion of natural capital may be increasing our healthcare costs. The more oblivious we are to all of this correlation, the greater will be our dilemma in the future.

THE PARADOX OF HEALTHCARE COSTS—THE NEED FOR A GRAND SOCIAL EXPERIMENT

This section will focus attention on the current dilemma with regard to healthcare costs faced by both the developed and the developing worlds. On one hand, healthcare costs are increasing in the developing world for somewhat different reasons than the developed world. The developing world is exporting its healthcare problems to the developed world and the developed world is exporting its healthcare problems to the developing world. Outlined below are several hypotheses that may require further research by social scientists.

Healthcare costs may be geometrically proportional to very high per capita consumption or very low per capita consumption. According to a new report from the Worldwatch Institute, a Washington, D.C.-based research organization, for the first time in human history, the number of overweight people rivals the number of underweight people, exactly 1.1 billion.[6] Both these groups suffer from malnutrition, a deficiency or an excess in a person's intake of nutrients and other dietary elements needed for healthy living. Gary Gardner and Brian Halweil, authors of the book, "Underfed and Overfed: The Global epidemic of Malnutrition, state, "The hungry and the overweight share high levels of sickness and disability and shortened life expectancies."[7] Both developed and developing nations are paying a high price for malnutrition. The World Bank estimates that hunger cost India between 3 and 9 percent of its GDP in 1996.[8] Moreover, obesity cost the United States 12 percent of the national healthcare budget in the late 1990s, or $118 billion, more than double the $47 billion attributable to smoking.[9] In developed countries, all too often we resort to technofixes like liposuction procedures that now average 400,000 per year. [10]

In the developing world, the very low per capita consumption is primarily due to extreme poverty that is a result of a large and a dense population. Both high population rates and poverty rates are aiding the spread of several forms of communicable diseases. Diseases that appeared subdued such as tuberculosis and malaria, are fighting back with renewed ferocity. Some, such as cholera and yellow fever, are striking in regions once thought safe from them. Deadly new diseases such as Ebola haemorrhagic fever, for which there is no cure or vaccine, are emerging in many parts of the world. At the same time, the sinister role of hepatitis viruses and other infectious agents in the development of many types of cancer is becoming increasingly evident. In an article written by Stephen S. Morse, Ph.D., of Rockefeller University, New York, entitled, "Factors in the emergence of Infectious diseases," the author identifies ecological, environmental, and demographic factors that have exacerbated the "emerging" infectious diseases. [11]

In an increasingly "smaller" world, where travel is common, where the immediacy of the television allows us to plagiarize lifestyles, both the developing and the developed world are engaged in an economic

enigma that increase healthcare costs. All problems are further exacerbated on a global basis due to falling water tables, deforestation, accelerating climate change, etc. Very few researchers seem to seek answers
to the following questions: "Why did we have 1,008 tornadoes in 1998
alone in the U.S.? Was this due to a climatic change? Maybe a thinning
of the ozone?" [12]

Several small scale "bottoms-up" social experiments can be carried
out by major agencies like the World Bank, United Nations Environment Program, local governments, industry, and by the people themselves. Developing countries need to address population reduction and
poverty alleviation strategies by entirely different methods than the
ones that are currently on vogue. These strategies may need to be built
around the total well being of human beings. Current policies in the
developing world do not seem to take into account the inherent talent
of people, possibly contributing to a greater desire to multiply, popu-
late urban areas, and a greater desire to accumulate short term wealth at
the expense of the environment.

Countries in the developing and the developed world may need to
pilot programs in specific regions of their countries that rely solely on
shifting an entire system from a one-time depletion of natural resources
to an economy that is based on a total replenishment of nature through
renewable energy, continuous recycling, and reuse of all materials. Systems of transportation should be completely converted to combina-
tions of foot, bicycle, or rail-based systems. Energy forms utilized must
be wind, solar and other such energy systems that are not invasive of
nature. The systems of education must switch from a culture of specialization to one that integrates knowledge into a collective vision. The
system of edifice construction and land construction may want to follow some of the traditional eastern philosophies that integrate the
methods of construction with the laws of nature, termed as *Feng-Shui*
in China and *Vasthu* in India. The EPA estimates that building-related
U.S. illnesses account for $60 billion of annual productivity lost

nationwide, and a wider study valued that loss as high as over $400 billion.[13]

The people in this experiment may want to switch to a plant—based diet. When the U.S. already has spent over $200 million in the Biosphere 2 experiment, there is no reason why a similar experiment cannot be revived. The Biosphere 2 experiment was a sunk cost and a forgotten research project, whereas the suggested experiments will not be a sunk cost, it would always serve as a living proof for generations to plagiarize. Life will still go on even if the experiment was abandoned.

Biosphere 2 was an experiment conducted in 1991, where eight scientists entered a sealed, glass-enclosed, 3.15 acre structure near Oracle, Arizona, where they remained for two years. Of the original 25 small vertebrae species introduced into the Biosphere, 19 became extinct. At the end of 17 months, because of the drops in oxygen levels, the humans were living in air whose composition was equivalent to a 17,500 foot altitude. It required $200 million and some of the best scientific minds in the world to construct a functioning ecosystem that had difficulty keeping eight people alive for 24 months. The Biosphere experiment showed that *human health is directly correlated with the natural state of health of the world:* the poorer the state of the ecological health, the higher will be our health costs. A perfect analogy that comes to mind that I borrow from eastern metaphysical thinking is that the macrocosm and the microcosm are structured the same. The trees are compared to the lungs of the earth; we destroy the trees, we destroy our own respiratory system. We destroy the skin of the earth (for example, the ozone) we destroy our own skin, the result of melanoma and other forms of skin cancer. We pollute the waters, we are polluting our own circulatory system with several infections and disorders of the circulatory system. A belief in these analogies is not only mystical and poetic, it shows how interconnected we are with the world.

These suggested experiments need to be designed through the involvement of the greatest thinkers in each of the countries of the world. We need thinkers who have humanistic impulses rather than thinkers whose impulses are geared for linear growth, generally through the exploitation of natural resources. If these experiments succeed, we should measure the total health outcomes of the people living in these kinds of colonies versus that of the average population. Only such experiments will challenge our thinking and will help the world evolve. Unless we develop diverse forms of economic systems, free choice in this world is a myth that parades in a single uniform.

All of these experiments do not undermine the scientific progress we have made in this world. Without some of the major contributions to medicine and several other scientific discoveries, our quality of life would have been far worse. We need parallel progress on all fronts in this world. Humanity will never follow any singular path, neither does it need to. We all have different tastes and belief systems. But, it is the burden of humanity to show a greater leaning towards technologies that do not deplete nature or even our natural state of well being. As we move forward, we certainly need a new paradigm of thought.

Unfortunately, the developing countries are at a more serious risk than the developed world. India is one-third the size of China and has more people per square mile than China. Both countries together account for 40% of the world population. What happens in these countries will reverberate across the world. Their problems will become the problems of the world. When the National Academy of Sciences recommended that China not adopt an automobile based system, they were simply ignored because these countries thought that they would be left behind in a global socio-economic race. China has ambitious plans to become a leading auto manufacturer. Unfortunately, sometimes the good intentions of America are sometimes confused because what America practices is sometimes different from what they preached. In the future, our foreign policy may gain more respect if it is shaped by institutions such as the Worldwatch Institute. In the U.S., we want to compete with the Eastern world with respect to their system of education which actually is styled after their western counterparts and has rapidly shifted to a "growth-based" education system that exploits nature and ecosystems. The root cause of most of our problems is a worldwide system of education that is based on "nature depleting technologies" rather than "nature replenishing technologies." The system of taxation on a worldwide basis is inconsistent and also lopsided.

In the words of Lester Brown of the Worldwatch Institute, "Today, at the dawn of a new century, faith in technology and human progress are as common as they were a century ago. In their fascination with information technologies, many of today's economic thinkers seem to have forgotten that our modern civilization, like its forerunners, is entirely dependent on its ecological foundations-foundations that the economy is now eroding." [14] Unless all systems of education all over the world address these issues, we may only exacerbate our problems. As a consequence, our solutions to healthcare will also be top-down.

The social innovations that I am talking about should not be confused with simple living. On the contrary, I am suggesting the conversion of all technologies from nature depleting to nature replenishing. The side effects of this approach could only be positive. It taps the inherent talent of people, improves well being, diminishes the gap between the rich and the poor and therefore lowers overall healthcare costs. *The greater the divide between the rich and the poor in society, the greater will be healthcare costs.*

Stephen Bezruchka, M.D., of the School of Public Health, University of Washington, has correctly pointed out that peoples' life span depends on the hierarchical structure of their society; i.e., the size of the gap between the rich and the poor. As economists know, the size of this gap is widening in both the developing and the developed world. Studies with baboons in Kenya and macaque monkeys in captivity, both of which feature strong hierarchical relationships, show that high-ranking animals are healthier than those in the lower pecking order. [15]

In 1960, Japan stood 23rd in the health olympic race, but by 1977 it had overtaken all the others in the health race. Today, at number 1, Japan has a life expectancy on average three and a half years longer than

United States.[16] Japanese CEOs make 15-20 times what entry-level workers make, not the almost 500-fold difference in this country.[17] Dr. Bezruchka, advocates a tax on consumption rather than income to diminish these gaps. Social experiments like the ones advocated here are complex and demand a grand vision. They do not fit well into the way we have been trained. The wrath of nature is no mystery. The better we treat nature and its all-inclusive systems, the better it will treat us. The mystery of healthcare costs will always remain intertwined in nature as well as, political, economic, and social systems. Perhaps it is the culmination of all these and several other factors that may be shaping our genes.

Summarized below is a quadrant diagram that provides a framework for healthy functioning for an individual, a society, an institution, a community, or even a country. The Y—axis of the quadrant shows the extreme situations of "values." These values relate to an individual, a company, a society, or a country. Similarly, the X-axis shows the two different extremes of attributes—"nature replenishing" or "nature depleting" with regard to the production and distribution of any product or service.

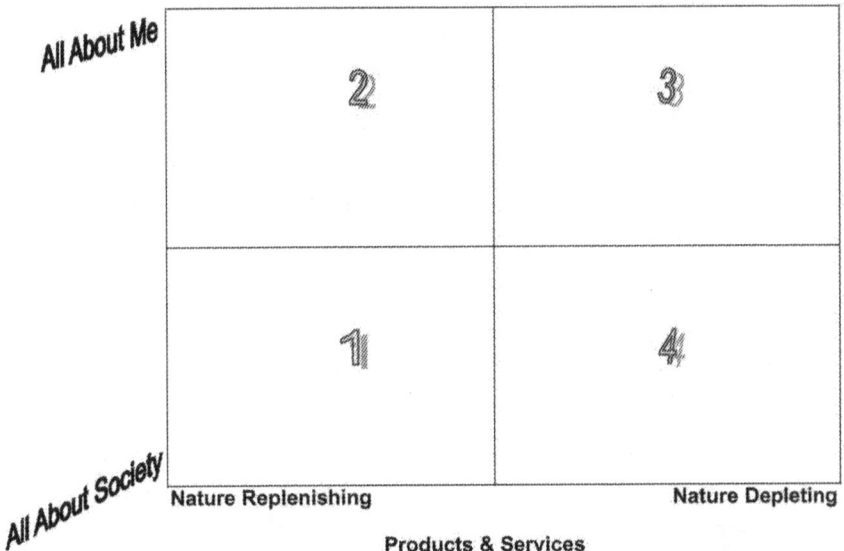

It is intuitive and logical that the more we focus on quadrant 3, the higher will be our costs of healthcare, the greater the gap between the rich and the poor, etc. Conversely, the more energy we spend in quadrant 1, the lower will be the costs of healthcare and the lower will be the gap between the rich and the poor.

This simple analytical tool will help shape individual, societal, and country specific policies. This tool not only addresses healthcare but it also addresses the health of our entire economic and social fabric. For example, the invention of electricity was "all about society." It narrowed the gap between the rich and the poor. Electricity as an invention when measured on the Y-axis could probably receive a score as high as a 5 (assuming a 0-5 scale). However, when electricity is measured on the X-axis, it could obtain a poor score, assuming a scenario in which electricity was produced by coal, hydroelectric, and fossil fuels only. Let us assume under such a scenario it got a score of 1. Therefore, the total score for electricity would be a 6. People might question my logic here since hydroelectric power is considered clean. Not true, when Alexander Gorlov served as a Soviet Adviser on Egypt's Aswan dam project four decades ago, he was astounded by the devastation the construction caused: 90,000 people were displaced and incalculable environment and arachaelogical damage was done.[18] Gorlov is now a Professor at Boston's Northeastern University and has developed the Gorlov Helical turbine that extracts power from water without requiring dams. It converts a streams kinetic energy into electricity with 35 percent efficiency than the 20 percent compared with conventional turbines.[19]

In this manner, when the governments all across the world evaluate their products and services, they could come up with tax criteria that are based on the consumption of goods and services as opposed to income. Tax criteria need to be developed based on pre-determined indices for each product and service produced in the economy. Products and services that have a very high index value will have a minimal tax, and products that have a low index value a very high tax. Under such an economic and tax framework, the incentive to develop and improve technologies will progress at a much more rapid pace. We may one day have computers that are biodegradable, plastic objects that replenish the soil, carpets that are biodegradable, etc. Fortunately several such technological innovations are already in existence but have never seen the light of the day since they threaten the existing business models of several companies. Most companies still seem to focus their energy on the Y-axis. The statements of vision and mission, ability to satisfy customers, as well as the competitive climate, seem to lend themselves to attain the right balance on the Y-axis. However, on a closer examination, we know most companies have probably done a poor job in terms of positioning themselves favorably on the X-axis. The closer organizations strive to reach the origin of the X and the Y-axis, the better positioned they will become to serve society and nature.

When a pharmaceutical drug is introduced into the human body, we evaluate the benefit to risk ratio. However, when inventions, products, and services are introduced into the cosmic body, we worry to a lesser degree about the benefit to risk ratios. Strategies for growth that move far away from the origin of X and the Y-axis eventually fail. These companies may provide a perception that they expand the economy while in the long term they only cause more harm than a benefit to the economy. The public may be skeptical of the likelihood of implementing such policies. In reality, they are not difficult if a phased approach is implemented, meaning a combination of taxes on income (our current state) and taxes on nature depleting technologies. It could also mean trying to first tax those products and services that have the most deleterious effects on the economy. Whichever scenario is implemented, the total tax rate should not exceed the current amount of tax paid collectively by all citizens. However, the suggested methods will narrow the disparities between the rich and the poor, thus ultimately impacting health in a favorable manner. As an alternative, we may also want to explore differential rates of capital gains taxation for people who invest in companies whose products and/or services replenish nature.

Once we understand all of the complex interrelationships of nature, health, environment and economics, we will be able to create a new era of leadership that is more balanced and harmonious. What is required is a model that challenges our current paradigm of thought, our current economic thinking, and the current system of education. Ideals, not strategies, should determine progress. When strategies determine progress, they often tend to be competitive. Total preoccupation in competitive acts and the so-called "winning-strategies" remove our focus on society. Our resulting actions, instead of helping, only end up harming the environment and the society in the long run. It is important that change start in small increments so that it causes the least disruption and allows institutions to adapt accordingly. Unless we start some small-scale experiments, there is no way to know what works and what do not.

THE CRITICAL NEED FOR A SMALL SCALE EXPERIMENT—WASTE AND HEALTHCARE COSTS

E-Waste—A practical illustration and a suggested approach may best describe the concepts stated above. I would like to focus on the e-waste phenomena that may be causing immense hazards to our health and how we can potentially rectify this situation. Transitioning from a nature depleting to a nature-replenishing scenario is certainly a viable option for the longer term. However, this should not stop us from seeking some practical solutions immediately.

"Although government regulation (of electronic waste) should come from the EPA (Environmental Protection Agency), the current administration hasn't seemed to go against industry much, particularly regarding environmental issues," said Scott Ribble, a policy associate at the non-governmental group Californians Against Waste (CAW).[20]

Electronic waste or E-waste consists of appliances ranging from refrigerators to stereos to sophisticated medical equipment, but personal computers pose the greatest threat because unlike most other appliances they become obsolete after an average of only two years. Computers contain cathode ray tubes (CRTs), like those used in televisions, which are coated in about four pounds of lead, as well as smaller amounts of other toxic materials such as arsenic and mercury, according to 'Poison PCs/Toxic TVs', a report by three California-based environmental groups—Silicon Valley Toxics Coalition (SVTC), Materials for the Future, and CAW. When personal computers that are dumped in landfills crack, the materials in them leach out and contaminate drinking water supplies and the air. Potential adverse effects from the 'e-waste' include DNA damage, asthmatic bronchitis, and mental retardation in children.[21] "Electronic waste is a very serious problem for three reasons," said Michael Alexander, a senior research associate at the non-governmental National Recycling Coalition. "Use of personal computers and other electronics is very widespread. Many of them have a very short life span. Many of them contain very toxic materials."[22] While 75 percent of obsolete computers remain stockpiled in homes and offices, the ones that are thrown out tend to come from households and small businesses rather than large corporations.[23]

The Resource Conservation and Recovery Act (RCRA), which became US federal law in 1999, makes American businesses—but not households—liable if they improperly dispose of hazardous waste such as CRTs. Large corporations that buy hundreds of computers every year tend to be more aware of RCRA laws than small businesses, and more willing to spend the money to recycle their machines, according to Alexander. Because households can legally dump their obsolete electronics in the trash, and because in all states but California and Massachusetts it is legal for municipal collectors to put CRTs in landfills, household computers often end up there.

Over 3.2 million tons of e-waste ends up in landfills every year.[24] Only 11 percent of computers discarded in the United States were recycled in 1999, according to a report by the National Safety Council, a non-governmental organization dedicated to helping people adopt practices that promote health and a clean environment.[25]

Hewlett-Packard, Gateway, Sony, IBM, Dell and Xerox are among manufacturers that already have take-back and recycling programs. Critics point out that most company-run recycling programs require consumers to pay a fee of 25 to 50 US dollars to recycle their obsolete electronics, and that they must also transport their machines to a recycling center themselves, making recycling unpalatable.

For all of these reasons, I recommend the following approach: Salvation Army or a Waste Management company open up e-waste disposal centers in their established locations all over the country. Salvation Army (or Waste Management companies through home-pick up) can then contract with a private company to ship them the old computers.

As demonstrated above, people do not want to go through the trouble of shipping their old computers to a specific destination—most people have no clue where these companies are located.

Recycling is a low margin business and hence companies may not aggressively advertise these services. What people need is a convenient drop-off zone since waste disposal companies who collect trash at houses may not pick up old computers. Therefore, I recommend Salvation Army consider this option as a means to fulfill a charitable cause and provide service to society. Most people would be willing to drop their computers at a Salvation Army facility close to their house for a nominal fee. Salvation Army itself can get into the business of e-waste recycling by employing local volunteer recruits from high schools. This would provide students much needed experience in assembling and ripping old computers apart. This can generate a new revenue stream for Salvation Army for its noble contributions to society. Alternatively, it can ship them to specific centers or even to the computer firms for a fee thus providing convenience and defraying customers from a more expensive shipping charge. Such partnerships between "not-for-profit" and the "for-profit" companies may be mutually beneficial.

Such an approach or a much more aggressive nationwide campaign is needed to educate consumers about the urgency of recycling electronics, and about the various ways to do it. Unless, these actions are pursued our healthcare costs may continue to increase.

Other Waste Related Innovations—There are several other related innovations that are urgently required in the area of waste management and waste disposal. For millenia, many cultures returned human waste to soils, and a few still do today. But increasingly the material is buried, incinerated, or flushed into rivers, bays, or oceans. The human toll for improper disposal (and from unclean water supply, often a related problem) is intolerably high: some 2 million children die each year and billions of people become sick because of inadequate water and sanitation facilities.[26] Universites in both the developing and the developed world need to design programs that teach organic and inorganic matter management as part of related degree programs. Degree programs in Business need to be more sensitive to human actions on ecology and ultimately their impact on health. Similarly, degree programs in agriculture need to be able to carry out inter-disciplinary research with medical professionals. For example, agricultural and medical professionals may conduct joint research on the overuse of manufactured fertilizers. The complete effects on health of manufactured fertilizers is yet to be understood. High levels of phosphorous and nitrogen in these fertilizers have promoted an overgrowth of algae in rivers, lakes and bays at the expense of other species, including various fish.[27] There is evidence that overuse of nitrogen and phosphorous can also be harmful to human health.[28] For all of the above reasons most degree programs need to integrate human interactions with the land they live in and how it ultimately impacts health. While most of us read magazines such as the Forbes, The Wall Street Journal, Money, etc., the focus of these magazines is on production and consumption. Not a single magazine aimed for the mass-market focuses attention on production, consumption, disposal, and the ultimate impact of technology and waste on the environment and human health. Our reading, thinking, and our educational training offers a totally one-sided picture of extraction, consumption, and a throw-way mentality. We all act as though there will not be a future generation. While we believe we are technologically sophisticated, we lack simple innovations of trashcans that distinguish between organic, inorganic, recycle, and e-wastes. While we have made improvements in distinguishing between plastics and paper (recycle waste) and non-recycle waste, several more simple home innovations are required that do not tax our landfills, oceans, seas, and air. As industries shift to zero-emission policies, so should consumers shift to zero-waste policies. This requires several unique innovations both on the industrial and the consumer front. We give more attention to the developing world when there is a financial meltdown in these regions and less attention when millions and billions of their lives suffer from industrial, automobile, and water pollution. We ignore the obvious and focus on the obscure. On the brighter side, the world has created a technical wonderland but on the darker side we have also created a technical wasteland. The greater the impact of the latter the greater the human suffering, tragedy, loss of lives and the increase in the costs of healthcare.

Thomas Berry, the most eminent cultural historian of our times presents the following as a challenge to human well-being, "In our view of a viable future, a new context would exist also for *the medical profession.* The problems of human illness are not only increasing but are being altered in their very nature by the industrial context of life. In prior centuries, human illness was experienced within the well being of the natural world with its abundance of air, water, and foods grown in fertile soil. Even city dwellers with their deteriorated natural surroundings could depend on the purifying processes of the natural elements. The polluting materials themselves were subject to natural decomposition and reabsorption into the ever-renewing cycles of the life process. But this in no longer true. The purifying process have been overwhelmed by the volume, the composition, and the universal extent of the toxic or non-biodegradable materials. Beyond all this, the biorhythms of the natural world are suppressed by the imposition of mechanistic patterns on natural processes."[29]

OTHER AVENUES FOR RESEARCH AND EXPERIMENTATION

What we learn from the ensuing paragraphs is the constant interplay and interaction between health, ecology, environment, and technology. This should lead us then to more carefully explore how we structure various professions and trades and how we ultimately design these processes into our educational system. For example, till the 17th century, in India, the carpenter was also the guardian of the forests. The ancient texts during those times abound in information regarding the types of trees that may be cut, the danger of over-felling, and the caution needed to keep the vegetation in its true state.[30] Similarly, the physician (known during those times as the *Vaidya*) not only looked after the sick and the healing but also helped in maintaining the hygiene, sanitation, diet, etc. for the healthy.[31] The architect likewise had the responsibility for the source of materials, depletion of forests, well-being of building related craftsmen, education and enlightenment of the common man/prospective clients, understanding and extending the functions of social metaphors and so on.[32] The relationship between the land and the human being was the essence of the organized community and the trades were structured accordingly. Practitioners in the various fields needed to have a basic knowledge and understanding of the traditions so that their action could always be appraised within the framework of human existence. Once our noble teaching institutions take up this challenge of researching land/human interactions and weave them into the several professional and degree programs, it is possible that one day it might have an impact on decreasing the phenomena of mental depression related to finding a meaning and value with work.

Summary

Perhaps while reading these seemingly disparate essays, one might conclude there is a lack of connectivity between all of the essays in this book. However, on closer introspection, all of these essays are indeed connected by a common theme: the lowering of healthcare costs through a balanced approach. The essays are an attempt to foster balance and harmony in a holistic manner rather than being tied to any political ideology.

Progress for most purposes is always equated with linear growth, the amount of products and services produced in the economy usually through the exploitation of natural and human resources. True progress is realized when high growth is accompanied by a replenishment of natural wealth, and associated well being of human lives with respect to their mental and physical states. When this does not happen, the general state of the health of a nation may suffer. Proof of this hypothesis lies in visiting institutions, regions, and countries where this happens to be true. This experience is more of internalization than a proof that needs a scholarly exposition.

The most preliminary and an obvious approach to healthcare reform may be a more "bottoms-up" approach that begins with defining an ideal that is wholesome to the individual and the society. It is this kind of approach that can compel us to think of personal responsibility and accountability. This approach is not the exclusive preserve of an individual, it applies equally to all of the variegated for-profit and not-for-profit institutions as well. When each of us acts without an ideal or a more parochially defined strategy, simply defined as being "All About Me," then imperfections in society begin to manifest themselves. It is the innumerable manifestations and varied hues of these self-centered actions that increase the costs of healthcare.

Unfortunately, most steps and measures adopted these days are to approach the crisis in healthcare from a top-down perspective. In some cases, top-down strategies make sense, but this again depends on context and practicality of application. For example, most physicians encourage tort reform to limit their medical liability costs. While the strategy is a top-down approach, it certainly may demand some merit. However, one should be careful in completely deviating away from a bottoms-up approach. Most top-down approaches tend to be intellectually pleasing and appear to be easily implementable, they automatically lend themselves to our traditional training, and satisfy the means of maintaining our livelihoods. Therefore, there is a greater tendency to lean on these approaches. "Top-down" and "Bottoms-up" each may have a rightful place. The acid test is how each approach increases or decreases societal well being, and increases or decreases the wealth of all mutually interdependent eco-systems. Seldom are such simulations discussed or debated.

A top-down strategy, without thought of its impact, may exacerbate the costs of healthcare. This is evident by the trajectory of the historical progress of nations when mapped to different types of disease states. For example, chronic diseases found among the poor in rural China may be different than chronic diseases found among the rich of Switzerland. Even within the same country, rich and poor may have different kinds of diseases. What is further surprising in most countries, including the U.S., is that the government itself does not think that they are in the business of promoting good health. On the contrary, when governments think and act as if they are not contributors of good health, but rather controllers of healthcare costs, they resort to approaches that tend to become top-down.

Similarly, organizations need to think of themselves as promoters of good health rather than institutions that are seeking to make health a complete business opportunity. When organizations promote good health as much as they cure a disease, they are truly replenishing natural resources. When healthcare organizations function in maintaining this kind of a balance sheet, they are less susceptible to the vagaries that arise due to the general criticism on the high costs of healthcare. While price and quality are the dominant criteria of any purchasing decision, free markets have not completely figured out on how to include environmental and health criteria into the purchasing decision of any product.

Educational institutions encourage and develop talent that fosters economic growth and fights competition. The emphasis of education is a focus on individual survival rather than the collective survival of individuals and their associated interactions with nature. As such, more energy is subconsciously spent on creating a workforce that drives consumption through the exploitation of scarce natural resources in an overpopulated world. These factors are further complicated by an ever widening gap between the rich and the poor. The immediacy of television and the superficial plagiarism of western technologies by the eastern nations have resulted in an adoption of cruder forms of technology in these countries. These technologies have totally disrupted the flora and fauna of these overpopulated nations. It is not that the technologies are at fault or the countries that even export or invent these technologies are at fault. It is the correct application of wisdom to apply these technologies that needs to be questioned. Plagiarism without context has exacerbated several forms of disease states directly attributable to the crude technologies and the associated disruption of the natural environment.

Despite the several seemingly obvious phenomena on environmental deterioration leading to poor health status, we tend to experiment ever more with newer technologies rather than retooling existing technologies that will replenish or not disrupt nature. While these technologies do have a place and benefit society, they are not the panacea for all our ailments. Solutions to healthcare may never come on a silver platter. In a society where over-consumption through the depletion of natural wealth has become synonymous with progress and extreme under-consumption with poverty and destitution, the manifestation of diseases reflect these very states of existence. Therefore, one must question both these states. While these essays try to harmonize the gravitational economic pull between the two halves of the world, they also emphasize the benefit of both halves of the world learning mutually about each others healthcare technologies. Within culture, context, and socio-economic background, each technology may thrive in its own right. Good health may only be achieved when individuals, institutions, and the government act in a concerted manner in a grand vision and an ideal that protects nature by constantly retooling existing technologies, questioning the current system of healthcare law, and applying technologies in the context of their social, cultural, and economic climate. Examples of these were covered in the many chapters of this book.

The purpose of any institution, government, or a country must be to nourish the lives of the millions of species in the earth's complex ecosystems. All of these species coexist in an intricate web of mutual interdependence and mutual enrichment. When individuals, institutions, and governments all over the world are oblivious to this interdependence, problems in health will arise. **Principles that support life directly influence the principles that govern life.** Therefore, the ideal must be to focus more on the former and less on the latter. It is the degree of focus in this world that is reversed and has tended to increase the global costs of healthcare. An approach that supports the basic principles that support life can be construed as being more "bottoms-up" than "top-down." The beginning and the ending chapters had some ideas on taxing consumption rather than income. I felt that this was a more practical way to negate the concepts of growth that do not replenish our natural wealth. This approach will not slow-down the free market economy. On the contrary, it will encourage more diverse forms of entrepreneurship. Free markets will be further challenged because existing business models may be threatened, but this is cleaner growth and cleaner competition. Civilizing and naturalizing capitalism through several innovative small-scale experiments may need to be encouraged. Appropriate identification of cause and effect phenomena may provide several clues to more wholesome progress. Such solutions may challenge the perfection of existing technologies and may simultaneously enhance our technological prowess. The very paradigms of economic cycles may be challenged, replaced by an economy that is more holistic. People like Amory Lovins have called this the creation of natural capitalism. Whether we like it or not, free markets will behave to maximize shareholder value through strategies that are either geared to satisfy a financial objective or occasionally a grander vision that truly benefits society. True ethics is simply not good behavior, but rather true ethics are about not causing harm to our environment through our products and services. This includes both living and the non-living beings. Certainly, America is more blessed than others for having created several checks and balances through compliance based laws such as the Clean Air Act, the Superfund, effective waste management techniques, etc., However, there is always room for improvement and innovation since the world watches us as a role model. Most countries do not have similar laws or similar infrastructure systems such as in America that support a healthier lifestyle. For this reason, these countries must be careful in how they implement globalization. This does not mean going backward in time or being frozen in time, but rather it means moving forward in time. For example, in one of my chapters I spoke about kinder, gentler hydroelectric power that does not necessitate the construction of dams. Such technologies are cheaper, better, and do not cause incalculable environmental or archaeological damage.

Radical changes cannot be achieved overnight. Change always begins with small and measured steps. Successful projects mostly grow from multiple small-scale experiments that mainly are an offshoot of a grand vision or an ideal. While some of the ideas in the essays may sound offensive to some people, they are not suggestive of a grand scale implementation. Grand scale schemes have always failed. Small-scale experiments simply provide answers to what works and what does not.

In systems that are complicated, we need to begin small, and if things work, broader implementation should be encouraged. Short-term benefits and living for today may sometimes appear more important than long-term benefits. A simple analogy here is the antipathy toward higher taxes on gas-guzzling cars or SUVs. Remember, it is the gas-guzzlers that primarily doubled the gasoline consumption over the last five years, thus raising price and disrupting the environment.[1] Yes, free markets work, a higher price on gas will work its way towards the development of a cleaner car. However, what we sacrifice in the bargain is the environment and the health, because economic forces tend to accelerate further exploitation of resources to bring prices down. Even the common layperson is aware of these everyday phenomena. These examples extrapolated on a grander scale have enormous implications that are further deleterious to health. Life, liberty, and the pursuit of happiness are the most precious gifts provided to us. However, they need to be accompanied by wisdom that does not cause harm to society and nature. Therefore, small-scale experiments may need to work on identifying the simple 80/20 rule, where twenty percent of our goods and services may be contributing to eighty percent of the deterioration of the health and the environment. The criteria may vary from one country to another. Moving forward, what may be required is an appropriate mix between taxes on consumption and taxes on income without raising the total current rate of taxation. Trying to shift the satisfaction of our heightened environmentally damaging consumption from the developed world to the developing world, which may manufacture all our plastic toys and all of our disposable products, will not solve the problem, it will only exacerbate the problem. Consumption in and of itself is not wrong, it is the damaging effects of consumption that needs to come under question. Simply speaking, any production process needs to take into account that the cycle of production, consumption, and non-nature replenishable waste is converted to a cycle of production, consumption, and replenishable waste. If every individual, industry, and nation walk on the former path, costs associated with healthcare will have to increase.

Certainly, I am not indicating that any of the experiments in this book are correct, other than to simply start a debate. What we are oblivious to in this world is the obvious connections between healthcare costs and the mechanistic view of the technological progress of this world. We are acting on a geological and biological order of magnitude. We are changing the chemistry of the planet. We are altering the great hydrological cycles. We are weakening the ozone layer, saturating the air, the water, the ocean, the fish, the fruits, the vegetables, and the soil with toxic substances so that we can never bring them back to their original state of purity. That the changes taking place are of this order of magnitude can be supported by reference to a conference held in September 1986 in Washington, D.C., a conference on the future of living species sponsored by the National Academy of sciences and the Smithsonian Institution. There our foremost biologists expressed forebodings concerning the future. Each of their statements shows the immense correlation between the environment and health.

At this conference, E.O. Wilson from Harvard indicated that we are losing ten thousand species each year and that this rate of loss is increasing. Norman Myers, a specialist in the rain forests and vegetation of the world, said that the "impending extinction spasm" is likely to produce the "greatest single setback to life's abundance and diversity since the first flickerings of life almost four billion years ago."[2] Other speakers agreed that our present extinction of living forms is, in its order of magnitude, paralleled only by the great geological and climatic upheavals that changed the earth in the distant past. In the words of Thomas Berry, a historian of cultures, "The natural world is subject as well as object. The natural world is the maternal source of our being as earthlings and the life-giving nourishment of our physical, emotional, aesthetic, moral, and religious existence. The natural world is the larger sacred community to which we belong. To be alienated from this community is to become destitute in all that makes us human. To change this community is to diminish our own existence."[3] Therefore, we can conclude that continued technological progress without regard to nature diminishes our very own existence, and may be first noticed as the rising costs of healthcare.

No matter how grand a vision, things will not change overnight. But we have to begin somewhere through small-scale bottoms-up experiments, several small-scale alliances, creative partnerships among several institutions, and most important, we must be willing to give things a try. Testing opposing ideas may only broaden our vision. Small-scale experiments will not stifle free markets, they certainly pose a challenge to existing business models. Therefore, they allow us opportunities to learn on what may work and what may not work. The thoughts and ideas in some of these essays may or may not be correct, but experiments certainly expand our vision. I do not profess to be an expert, I am a lay person who wants his opinion heard. But there is no denying the fact that principles that support life need to be our focus; if we truly want to contain the costs of healthcare. If we are losing ten thousand species each year, we cannot deny the truth that in some way it is affecting our own lives as well.

The profession of medicine and all other professions must now consider their role, not only within the context of human society, but also in the context of the Earth process. Our educational institutions, our government, and our industry need to take the lead to establish a way of sustaining the species as well as the individual if the human is to be viable as a species within the community of species.

In summary, a committed appreciation for all processes that support human and non-human life (i.e., all ecosystems in the world) are the primary means to lowering our long-term healthcare costs. There are several other secondary approaches that will lower our short-term healthcare costs. A few that were listed in this book related to : creating diverse and unique preventive health models, a more bottoms-up cause and effect analysis of patent laws, medical education, evaluation of taxation and economic systems, immediate impact of major technological innovations on human health, innovations in the medical field that encourage diversity of thought, lowering costs through product, process, and commonsense innovations. The most important innovation will have to come from Schools and Universities (all across the world) to incorporate ecological thought process into every field of endeavor.

Bibliogaphy

PART 1: Chapter 1
Innovations in Preventive Health

1. Cowley, G., "How to Live 100." *Newsweek*, June 30, 1997, pp. 57-67

2. Ibid

3. Ibid

4. Liebmann, O., "Blueprint for Managed Foodcare." *The Wall Street Journal*, July 18, 1994

5. "News Bytes." *The Pharmaceutical Executive*, September 2000, p 166

6. Ibid

7. **http://www.tnty.com/press/transcripts**

8. Heper, M., "Biotech Corn Leads to a Series of Recalls." A News Release on **http://www.forbes.com/**

9. Hayden, T., "A Growing Coral Crisis." *Newsweek*, Oct 30, 2000, pp79

10. Patz, J.A., "Need for Expanded Scope of Occupational and Environmental Medicine." *Climate Change and Health*, (From an excerpt of the book publication on the EPA Global Warming website)

11. Henry, S., "Are you Completely Inactive? Moderate, Vigorous, Regular—What does it mean?" *(From* **http://www. fitnesslink.com/exercise/moderate.shtml***)*

12. "Reward Health with Wealth," *(From* **http://www. fitnesslink.com/info/tax.shtml***)*

13. Ibid

14. Kummer, B., "Ignore Heartburn at your own Risk." Fall Health and Fitness Section of *The Newsweek,* Oct 16, 2000, p14

15. In the News Section of "Did you Know." *Popular Science*, March 2001, p 70

16. See note 1

17. See note 1, page 59

PART 1: Chapter 2
The Medicaid Food Stamp Program—A Novel Experiment in Preventive Health

1. "Drop in Food Rolls is Mysterious and Worrisome." *The Wall Street Journal*, Monday, August 2, 1999, page A20

2. "$1.8 billion eaten in food stamp bilks." *The Star Ledger*, Monday, July 18, 1994, page 3

3. Senauer, B., "America's Second Currency: A Staple for 1 in 10 Food Stamp Program may Face Reforms." *The Region*, 1993 (http://minneapolisfed.org/pubs/region/93-03/reg933b.html)

4. Position of The American Dietetic Association: The Role of Nutrition in Health Promotion and Disease Prevention Programs. *J Am Diet Assoc*. 1998;98:205-208

5. American Cancer Society. 1996 Guidelines on Diet, Nutrition and Cancer
   Prevention.

6. Prescription Drug Expenditures and Projections for 2002-2010 was listed on the HCFA website

7. In 1999, the total dollar outlay on the Medicaid Food Stamp program was about $15.8 million based on USDA statistics on the USDA website. Year 2010 projection was estimated by the author.

PART 2: Chapter 3
Innovations in Healthcare
Strategy and Implications on
Healthcare Costs

1. Listed on the HCFA website (now called CMS). Check for Table 1: National Health Expenditures and Selected Economic Indicators, Levels, and Average Annual Percent Change: Selected Calendar Years 1970-2008.

2. Ibid. See Table 2

3. National Vital Statistics Report, Vol. 47, No. 28, December 13, 1999. Available on the web.

4. The Future of Healthcare: A Harvard Magazine Roundtable. Listed on the web **http://www.harvard-magazine.com/issues/ma99/healthcare.html**

5. Ibid

6. Ibid

7. "Well Being Improves for Most Older People, But Not for All." *NIH News Release*, Aug 10, 2000. (See **http://www.nih.gov/nia/news/pr2000/**

8. Walters, W.C. III., *The Grand Disguise.* A Press Release on the Book from Amazon.com

9. Offitt, P.A., and Bell, L.M., *What Every Parent Should Know about Vaccines.* See Chapter 1, page3. Macmillan USA, 1998.

10. Reid, W.V., and Miller, K.R., "Keeping Options Alive: The Scientific Basis for Conserving Biodiversity." listed on the website of the World Resources Institute, 1989.

11. Ibid

12. Fisher, A., "Dangerous Gas." *Popular Science*, December, 2000.

13. Colburn, D.T., Dumanski, D., and Myers, J.P., *Our Stolen Future: Are We Threatening our Fertility, Intelligence, and Survival,* Penguin Books, New York, 1996.

14. Plotkin, M., *Medicine Quest: In Search of Nature's Hidden Cures*, Viking Publishers, New York, 2000.

15. Artuso, A., "Natural Product Research and the Emerging Market for Biochemical Resources." *Journal of Research in Pharmaceutical Economics*, Vol. 8 (2). 1997.

16. See note 14

17. Christensen, C.M., Bohmer, R., and Kenagy, J., "Will Disruptive Innovations Cure Healthcare." *Harvard Business Review*, September—October 2000. See pages 13-110

18. Krucoff, C., "The Best Anti-Stress Medicine May be Right under Your Nose," *Washington Post,* May 2, 2000.

19. Rosenfeld, I., "The New Short Term Antibiotics," *Parade Magazine*, Jan 28, 2001, page 11

20. Michael, O., "Doctor Creates a Rift with a Radical Notion: Prescribe Fewer Pills," *The Wall Street Journal*, Friday, June 22, 2001, pp A1

21. Research News and Opportunities in Science and Theology, November, 2000, Vol. 1, No. 3. (Published by the Templeton Foundation)

22. Ibid

23. See note 14; page 201. Also, see: La Barre, W., "Hallucinogens and the Shamanic Origins of Religion," *In Flesh of the Gods*, Allen & Urwin, London, 1972. See pages 261-278.

24. Hawken, P., Lovins, A., & Lovins, H., *Natural Capitalism: Creating the Next Industrial Revolution*, Rocky Mountain Institute. See pages 70-71. Also see: **http:/www.rmi.org**

25. See article on "Patient Centered Healthcare: The Road to Wellville," This is a publication of The Citizens Against Government Waste (CAGW) and is available on the website at **http://www.cagw.org/publication**

26. The Year 2000 Annual Report of CISCO

PART—2: Chapter 4
Some Innovations in Information Technology that will Lower Healthcare Costs

1. See article on "Patient Centered Healthcare: The Road to Wellville," This is a publication of The Citizens Against Govern-

ment Waste (CAGW) and is available on the website at **http:// www.cagw.org/publication**

2. Ibid

3. Landro, L., "Web Health Groups Ponder How to set Universal Standards," *The Wall Street Journal*, Friday, November 3, 2000.

4. Boisclair, M "In the Palms of their Hands" *Pharmaceutical Executive*, September 2000, pp. 154-158Journal, Friday, November 3, 2000

5. Ibid

6. "Finding the Right Rx" *Newsweek*, pp. 66-67, September 20, 1999

7. News item on Bill Sharpe, *Worth*—Magazine, October, 2001, page 100

8. Korten, D., "Enemy of the People: Modern Capitalism's Triumph is not a Victory for Democracy." *Forbes ASAP*, October 4, 1999, pp. 118

9. Ibid

10. Ibid

11. Ibid

PART—3: Chapter 5
Innovations in Policy and Reform that may Lower Healthcare Costs

1. Cloud, J., "A Kinder and Gentler Death." *Time*, September, 18, 2000. pp. 61-67

2. Ibid

3. Ibid

4. Ibid

5. Vida Foubister, "Medical Experts Agree on Guide for End-of-Life Care." *American Medical News*, Volume 43, Number 5, Feb 7, 2000.

6. Frankenfield, G., "Cell Phone Use While Driving Increases Risk." *WebMD Medical News*, Feb 24, 2000. See: **http://www.webmd.lycos.com**

7. O'Neill, J.E., "Medicine and Graduate Medical Education." Listed on **http://www.cbo.gov/** A September 1995 Bulletin.

8. See Note 1

9. Braus, P., "Women and Medicine". **http://web.gmu.edu/departments/safe/r-world/wofw/femmed.html** 1994

10. "The American Health Care System—Physicians in the Changing Marketplace." New England Journal of Medicine, Volume 340 Number 7, Feb 18, 1999. Page 587

11. Ibid

12. Ibid

13. Ibid

14. Ibid

15. Knox, A., "New Drugs Bringing Questions and Recalls." *The Philadelphia Inquirer*, Sunday, January 7, 2001.

16. Ibid

17. See article on "Patient Centered Healthcare: The Road to Wellville," This is a publication of The Citizens Against Government Waste (CAGW) and is available on the website at **http://www.cagw.org/publication**

PART—3: Chapter 6
Re-engineering Medicare—An Approach to its Solvency

1. Iglehart, J.K., "The American Health Care System—Medicare," *New England Journal of Medicine*, Jan 28, 1999, Volume 340, 327-332. Also, see **http://www.medicare.gov**

2. Ibid

3. Ibid

4. Ibid

5. Ibid

6. Brown, R., and Gold, M., "What drives Medicare Managed care Growth," *Health Affairs*—Volume 18, Number 6, pp. 140-148

7. Ibid

8. Ibid

9. "Kaiser Takes the Cyber Cure." *Business Week*, February 7, 2000, PP EB80-EB94

10. Anders, G., "Dealing with Data: Companies have lots of high-tech ideas for improving how doctor's and hospitals handle medical

information." *The Wall Street Journal*, Monday, October 19, 1998. Page R25

11. Ibid

12. A Sachs/Scarborough Healthplus Survey listed on **www. connect.claritas.com/Doc/OSPsample.htm**l

13. See Note 9

14. See Note 9

15. See Note 12

16. Bodenheimer, T., "Long Term care for Frail Elderly People—The On Lok Model," *The New England Journal of Medicine*, Oct 21, 1999, Vol. 341, No 17, 1327

PART 4: Chapter 7
Stress, Organizational Design, and Long Term Effects on Health and Costs

1. United Nations International Labor Organization, "Stress at Work," in *World labor Report 6, United Nations International Labor Office*, Geneva, Switzerland, 1993

2. Brothers, J., "You Can Lead a More Joyful Life." *Parade Magazine*, October 15, 2000, pp 6-7

3. Ibid

4. *Research News and Opportunities in Science and Theology*, February 2001, Vol. 1, No. 6.

   Page 7. (Published by The Templeton Foundation, Durham, NC)

5. Bill Joy's statement at a seminar, see *Worth magazine*, June 2000. p29

6. *Research News and Opportunities in Science and Theology,* November 2000, Vol. 1, No. 3.
    Page 9. (Published by The Templeton Foundation, Durham, NC)

PART 4: Chapter 8
Balancing Technological Progress with Social Innovations to contain Healthcare Costs

1. Ehrlich, P., *Human Natures : Genes, Cultures, and the Human Prospect,* Island Press / Shearwater Books, California, 2000) pp 328-329

2. Golder, L., and Heal, G., "Do We Overconsume?" Chocolate Group Seminar, Center for Conservation Biology, Stanford University Press, 5 March 1999

3. Hawken, P., Lovins, A., & Lovins, H., *Natural Capitalism: Creating the Next Industrial Revolution,* Rocky Mountain Institute. See: **http:/www.rmi.org**

4. Ibid

5. See Note 1 pp289-290

6. "Chronic Hunger and Obesity Epidemic Eroding Global Progress." A Worldwatch News Release, Worldwatch Institute, Washington, D.C., 4 March 2000 See: **http:/www. worldwatch.org/alerts**

7. Ibid

8. Ibid

9. Ibid

10. Ibid

11. Morse, S.S., "Factors in the Emergence of Infectious Diseases," *EID,* Volume 1, Number 1, Jan—March 1. **http://www/cdc.gov/ ncidod/edi/vol1no1/morese.html**

12. See "Note From a World Watcher ; Specialization and Tunnel Vision." *Worldwatch Magazine,* Sep/Oct 1999. See: **http:/www.worldwatch.org/mag**

13. See Note 3. Chapter 5, pp 88-89

14. "New Century to be marked by growing threats, opportunities." *A Worldwatch News Release; State of the World 1999.* Worldwatch Institute, Washington, D.C., See: **http:/www/worldwatch.org**

15. Bezruchka, S., "Is Our Society making you Sick," *Newsweek,* February 26, 2001. pp14

16. Ibid

17. Ibid

18. *Popular Science,* December 2001. pp 26

19. Ibid

20. Biet, L., "Old Computers a Toxic Bomb," A news item that appeared on the Malyasiakini.com. See **http://www. malyasiakini.com/News**

21. Ibid

22. Ibid

23. Ibid

24. Ibid

25. Ibid

26. Brown, L.R., Flavin, C., French. H., *State of the World 1998*, A Worldwatch Institute Report on Progress Toward a Sustainable Society. pp 101

27. Ibid p 99

28. Ibid p 100

29. Berry, T., *The Great Work : Our Way Into the Future*, Bell Tower, New York, pp 66-67

30. Ananth, S., printed from

   http://www.fengshuiseminars. com/articles/Tradition%20and%20Modernity.html

31. Ananth, S., printed from

   http://www.fengshuiseminars. com/articles/sacredarchitecture.html

32. Ibid

Summary

1. Easterbrook, G., "Toward a Sound Oil Policy." On **http:// www.middle-east-online.com/English/Opinion**. Also, **http:// www.sierraclub.org/globalwarming/cleancars/cafe/ gasprices.asp**

2. Berry, T., *The Dream of the Earth,* Sierra Club Nature and Natural Philosophy Library, San Francisco, CA. 1988. pp 354-356

3. Ibid (see quote on cover jacket)

About the Author

Ram Ramprasad works in a management capacity for a healthcare related company. He has worked in the healthcare industry for 15 years. Ram held a wide variety of positions in his career. Prior to entering the healthcare field, he consulted at American Cyanamid and held a logistics position with a trading company in New York. Before he came to the U.S. for his graduate studies, he lectured undergraduate business students at Bayero University in Nigeria and designed programs for executives.

Ram received a Master of Business Administration degree from Madras University in India. He is also a graduate in International & Economic Development from Yale University. He lives on the East Coast with his wife and two children.

0-595-24167-0

www.ingramcontent.com/pod-product-compliance
Lightning Source LLC
Chambersburg PA
CBHW061249280526
45784CB00002B/701